10-MINUTE
YOGA
WORKOUTS

POWER TONE YOUR BODY
FROM TOP TO TOE

Barbara Currie

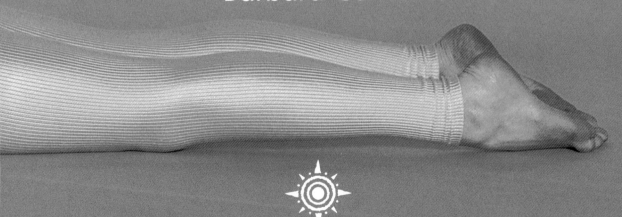

Thorsons

To my wonderful family: my mother Babs, my husband Gordon, my children Lysanne and Mark, and my brother Richard with many thanks for your unconditional love and support.

Thorsons
An imprint of HarperCollins*Publishers*
77–85 Fulham Palace Road,
Hammersmith, London W6 8JB

The Thorsons website address is: www.thorsons.com

and *Thorsons*
are trademarks of HarperCollins*Publishers* Limited

First published 2002

10 9 8 7 6 5 4 3 2 1

© Barbara Currie 2002

Barbara Currie asserts the moral right to
be identified as the author of this work

Photography by Guy Hearn

A catalogue record of this book
is available from the British Library

ISBN 0 00 712961 0

Printed and bound in Italy by
Editoriale Johnson SpA

Not all exercises are suitable for everyone. To reduce the risk
to you, please consult your doctor before beginning this
exercise programme. The instructions and advice presented are
in no way intended as a substitute for medical guidance. The
writer and publishers of this book do not accept any responsi-
bility for any injury or accident as a result of following this
exercise programme.

contents

acknowledgements

I would like to thank: Wanda Whiteley for her enthusiasm and encouragement and for making this book possible; Samantha Grant for all her help and creative ideas with our photoshoot; Simon Gerratt; Matthew Cory for his wonderful work in editing my initial script; Guy Hearn for his brilliant photography and his patience and help with the photoshoot; Sallyann Sexton for my beautiful make-up and hair-dressing in impossible positions; Polly Zabari for typing my script and meeting all my deadlines with a big smile – despite giving birth halfway through the book; Julie Drakeford-Lewis, Kelly Defoy, Claire Mullins and Jay Ridout, my yoga A-Team, for posing so beautifully for the illustrations in this book; and Joanne Cassidy for her patience and help during the photoshoot; Natasha Fidler for her beautiful page design and Sonia Dobie for the wonderful cover.

introduction

I'll never forget my first yoga class. It was one grey dreary Monday morning that I ventured inside a hall on the outskirts of Glasgow, and enrolled for yoga lessons. At that time I felt tired, stiff, out of shape and frazzled, due to having just moved house with two children under the age of 3. I had only a vague idea about yoga but thought that it might help me reshape my body after the birth of my children, and also help me to get to know my new neighbours.

It was an incredibly humbling experience, I couldn't believe how stiff and uncoordinated I was, I was only 29 but people twice my age were in much better shape and much more flexible than me. My biggest shock was seeing my teacher, then in her late fifties, move effortlessly into seemingly impossible positions with the agility of a child. Her body was fantastic – she was slim and perfectly toned – but it wasn't just this that amazed me; it was something much, much more. She had an energy that literally radiated from her, lighting up the room.

I left the class feeling so much better, my tiredness had gone, I felt calmer and more in control. I was walking taller and felt uplifted by the experience. One thing was certain – yoga was definitely for me. As I continued with the classes, I was thrilled by the progress I was making, my body had become firmer, my flexibility had improved and my energy level was getting better and better.

Eventually I decided to take a three-year teacher training course and this gave me a fantastic understanding of yoga, its history, philosophy and many uses. Over the years I have continued to study and teach yoga at my yoga school in Surrey and I have taught literally thousands of pupils. I have now perfected my own method of teaching which, I feel relates this brilliant 5,000-year-old system to the needs of people living today.

I am delighted to have this wonderful opportunity of sharing it with you. I do hope you will enjoy it and will benefit tremendously from its age-old secrets.

A Brief Word About Yoga

The word yoga means union of body, mind and spirit with the universal spirit. The yogis of ancient India realized that for perfect health and inner peace, both body and mind must work together in perfect harmony. Yoga's combination of intricate physical postures, deep breathing exercises, balances, relaxation and meditation are the perfect discipline to relieve stress, calm the mind and tone the entire body, both inside and out.

In his quest to earn more, do more and have more, modern man subjects himself to increased physical and mental stress. The pace of life is now so fast that few of us have time to enjoy the present moment and just be.

Continued stress on both body and mind increases our vulnerability to disease. Unfortunately, although medicine has made many amazing breakthroughs in the West over the last hundred years, the focus continues to be on treating diseases and not their causes. This is where yoga can help us all so much. Stress or tension literally strangles our bodies, inhibiting blood flow to our tissues. Yoga's beautiful physical movements, combined with deep breathing exercises, will carefully rid the body of tension and stimulate oxygen-rich blood to our cells, so providing them with the nutrients that they require. As well as toning all our muscles, the physical exercises will also strengthen our bones and keep our spine and joints flexible. The lymphatic system, which fights infection and carries away toxins, is inhibited during times of stress, but as yoga carefully smoothes away the tension, it can resume its natural functions.

Yoga's calming balances necessitate tremendous concentration and so they take the mind off its day-to-day activities, giving it a rest. The most difficult thing to discipline, however, is the human mind. Here again yoga offers us many techniques, from breathing exercises to relaxation and meditation, which may be used to calm a turbulent mind. Gradually and with continued practise the combined discipline of the exercises together with the breathing and meditation will help us to achieve the peace and calm we desire. And just as stress inhibits our energy flow, a calm and peaceful mind will lead to abundant energy and that genuine 'good to be alive' feeling.

Eventually, we stop looking elsewhere for our pleasures and concentrate on 'looking within', disciplining our mind to search inside ourselves for our joy and happiness. We then start to enjoy the present moment, and listen to our gut instincts, finally achieving self-realization and finding the true health and happiness that is within us all.

THE ORIGINS OF YOGA

It is unclear when yoga actually originated, but seals were discovered depicting a yoga posture during the excavation of some ruins in prehistoric India in an area that now lies in Pakistan. These ruins revealed a very advanced civilization dating to around 5000BC.

The earliest texts mentioning yoga were the Vedas, and these seem to have spanned about 2,000 years, from 3000–1200BC. These texts were followed by the Upanishads, written between 800 and 400BC. The word Upanishad literally describes a sitting where the master or guru instructs his pupils. This is how yoga has been passed on from generation to generation, over the years. The spirit of the Upanishads can be compared with that of the New Testament 'The Kingdom of God is within you'.

'Meditation is a truth higher than thought. The earth seems to rest in silent meditation; and the waters and the mountains and the sky and the heavens seem all to be in meditation. When a man achieves greatness on this earth, he has his reward according to his meditation.'

CHANDOYA UPANISHAD 7.6

The Bhagavad Gita, dating from about 500BC, tells of the struggle of the human soul, helping it to find God in all things and all things in God. It tells of a great battle for the rule of a Kingdom or the Kingdom of the soul, a battle between the forces of light and darkness. It shows that this is a battle that affects us all.

The Patanjalis Yoga Sutras, written between 200BC and 200AD, are a crucial yoga text. Patanjali wrote of a practical eight-part approach to yoga, frequently referred to as the Eight Limbs of Yoga.

'Restraint, observance, posture, breath-control, sense withdrawal, concentration, meditative-absorption and enstasy are the eight members of yoga.

Non-harming, truthfulness, non-stealing, chastity and greedlessness are the restraints.'

PATANJALIS YOGA SUTRAS II, 29–30

These eight limbs were not regarded as a ladder to be climbed one rung at a time, but more the necessary ingredients in the recipe for life. The ancient yogis realized that life can be a difficult and complicated journey but its careful teachings and disciplines guide us along our path. They had a deep understanding of man's nature and of the mind–body connection, and they devised this system to help us obtain happiness and peace of mind, as well as a perfectly toned healthy body.

The Eight Limbs of Yoga

1 Yamas

These are guidelines necessary for our moral conduct and are the basic principles of right living and restraint; they are no violence, stealing or envy and they command us to be truthful with both others and ourselves. Yoga teaches us that happiness is not in external objects but within ourselves and that the spirit of God is within each one of us.

2 Niyamas

These are the personal disciplines of daily life. They are cleanliness of mind and body, purity, contentment, study, work and devotion to God or the universal spirit. Yoga teaches us that the body is the temple of the spirit and keeping the body in perfect condition is our duty.

3 Asanas

These are the yoga exercises or postures. It is said that there are 840,000 of them! These movements work the entire body, freeing it from tension, toning and firming and strengthening every muscle, internal organ and gland. The balancing postures teach us the power of concentration and focus. Deep relaxation calms the mind and rids the body of chronic tension, and meditation trains the mind to achieve stillness and peace.

4 Pranayama

This is yoga's breath control. There are many breathing exercises in yoga to stimulate life-giving oxygen to every cell, to energize the body and calm and soothe the mind. The word pranayama means 'controlling the energy flow'. Yoga teaches us how to use our breathing to control our life.

5 Pratyahara

This is the withdrawal of the senses from the external world to the self within to give one peace and calm. This is achieved by practising the asanas and pranayama. Most of our daily activities necessitate our concentration and involvement with external objects and thoughts, but by concentrating on our body as we do the movements, and by concentrating on our breathing, the mind and body become peaceful and calm.

6 Dharana

This is the power of constant concentration and focusing of the mind. The mind is like the rays of the sun. When spread over a wide surface, the rays will be warming, but concentrate the rays and they become powerful enough to burn. Yoga balances start us on this path. They discipline the mind to concentrate on just one spot while performing the balances. This skill develops so that eventually one is able to concentrate and focus on a subject of interest even in the midst of turmoil.

7 Dhyama

This is meditation. Meditation is a powerful tool for freeing our minds from the pressures of life, helping us feel peaceful and calm. When this is accomplished, new ideas appear and the way ahead looks clearer.

8 Samadhi

This is the result of our total efforts and is the experience of enlightenment and bliss, living in the present moment, and the realization that we can manifest whatever we wish. The mind becomes full of joy and peace. It is the state of union with the universal spirit or God.

Another very important yoga text is the Hatha Yoga Pradipika, written by Svatmarama in the 16th century. The legend of the origin of this book is as follows:

> *'Goddess Parvati, the wife of Lord Siva approached her Lord – the seed of all knowledge for guidance to ease all the sufferings of humanity. Lord Siva then revealed to her the greatest of all sciences for the holistic development of man – the science of hatha yoga.'*
>
> B.K.S. IYENGAR

This knowledge was then passed on from guru to pupil until, eventually, Svatmarama wrote it down in the Pradipika. Hatha Yoga is the yoga most commonly practised in the West today. It is the physical aspect of yoga. The aim is to perfect the health of the body and mind by physical exercises, balances, deep relaxation, meditation and breath control, and dietary observances.

> *'Anyone who actively practises yoga be he young, old or even very old, sickly or weak can become a siddha [obtain yoga benefits and powers]. Anyone who practises can acquire siddhis, but not he who is lazy. Yoga siddhis are not obtained by merely reading textbooks.*
>
> *'Nor are they reached by wearing yoga garments, or by conversations about yoga, but only through tireless practise. This is the secret of success. There is no doubt about it.'*
>
> HATHA YOGA PRADIPIKA CH4, V64–66

Yoga Today

The collective knowledge of these ancient texts began to appear in the West at the end of the nineteenth century and since then interest in yoga has grown and today it is at an all time high. Students of all ages are pouring into classes to learn yoga, and for many diverse reasons. Some come simply to improve their body shape, some to cure an aching back, some to relieve stress. Whatever the reason, yoga can help you live healthily in this chaotic, exciting and wonderful modern world.

While Hatha yoga remains the most widely practised form of yoga in the West, other forms include:

○ Raja Yoga – the yoga of the mind;
○ Karma Yoga – the yoga of action;
○ Bhakti Yoga – the yoga of devotion;
○ Jhana Yoga – the yoga of the intellect.

Because of the many approaches to teaching yoga, finding a class to suit you can be very confusing. I often receive phone calls from people inquiring as to what sort of yoga I teach. I suppose that since I have been teaching for over 30 years, by now I have put my individual stamp on the ancient art. Throughout this time, I have tried to make yoga understandable, enjoyable and available to everyone. It is my firm belief that everyone can benefit tremendously from yoga practise.

But how can you find a class that will be to your liking? I am afraid that this will be a bit like trying to find everything else – from a plumber to a dentist. Often you have to try several until the perfect one appears. There are some excellent yoga teachers around, quite simply search for a class until you find one that works for you. As a first move, you can't do better than look in your local newspaper to find classes running near where you live.

Guidelines for Practising Yoga

You need very little equipment for your yoga practise so it is easy to fit in with any lifestyle. Once you have learnt your basic movements you can do them at home or on holiday. Your yoga will go with you wherever you go. Having said this, there are a few basic guidelines that you should take note of before you start.

o You need a warm airy room if you are practising inside, but in warmer climates it is wonderful to do your yoga in the fresh air in the warmth of the early morning or evening. Never practise in the heat of direct sun.

o You need a mat or blanket to sit on. My preference is for a blanket or thick warm mat for internal practice. However, if you are practising yoga outside, perhaps on a beach, you need a waterproof mat to keep you clean and dry.

o Wear loose clothing, ideally a leotard and leggings for women, or leggings and a close fitting t-shirt. Jogging bottoms or shorts and a t-shirt are best for men. If you are outdoors in a warm climate, your swimsuit is just fine.

o Bare feet are essential for yoga practice.

o Always wait at least two hours after a main meal before you practise yoga.

o **The golden rule of yoga is never ever to strain.** Don't worry if you are stiff and uncoordinated to start with. This is quite normal. Just persevere, work at your own pace and you will be delighted at how quickly your body responds to the movements and how much more flexible you are after only a few weeks of practise. You will start to feel better almost immediately and will soon be delighted with your new svelte shape.

o Although yoga is for everyone, if you have any health concerns it is always wise to check with your doctor before you begin.

○ **Never substitute yoga for your doctor's treatment.** Yoga is good for your health and some movements are particularly beneficial for certain conditions. However, they must never be substituted for your doctor's treatment.

○ **Yoga and pregnancy.** If you are pregnant and have not done any yoga before, then please wait until after your check-up at about 15 weeks. If everything is OK and your doctor is happy, then you may start to practise yoga very gently, omitting the movements marked unsuitable for pregnancy. (For more on this, see page 173).

○ **Following the baby's birth.** Wait until after your six-week check-up before you recommence your yoga practice. If your doctor is happy for you to recommence your yoga practice, then inform your teacher of the nature of your delivery. Go gently and soon you will find your shape and energy coming back fast.

○ **Breathing.** In yoga, we breathe deeply with every movement to help to stimulate oxygen to every cell, and energize our entire systems. Breathing is done through the nose. As a general rule, gently allow your abdominals to push out as you inhale deeply through the nose at the start of a posture and exhale slowly and quietly through the nose as you go into the movement. While in the positions, breathe calmly and peacefully through the nose.

Using This Book

PART 1

Having studied and taught yoga for nearly 30 years, I have spent a lot of time listening to my pupils and realize that only a lucky few have time to do an hour's yoga a day. This is why the chapters in Part 1 of this book are set out as 10-minute sequences.

Chapters 1 and 2 – These offer a choice of Ten-minute Miracles, one for beginners and one for more advanced pupils. I would like you to start every day with one of these. They will keep your spine and joints really strong and flexible while toning virtually every muscle in your body. They are a wonderful energizing start to the day.

After this, fit Chapters 3–6 into your schedule to suit your own individual requirements and time available. One chapter a day would be great. If you do have time, even just once a week, to do all six 10-minute chapters, then that would give you a perfect balanced work-out for mind and body.

Chapter 3 – This sequence concentrates on yoga balances. These tone and firm and strengthen every muscle in the legs and bottom. They also teach us the power of concentration and focus and help us clear and concentrate the mind.

Chapter 4 – is magical for toning the thighs and bottoms, and really delivers results. It is also great for smoothing out cellulite.

Chapter 5 – This is your abdominal sequence. It really tones and firms the abdominals and slims the midriff and the waistline.

Chapter 6 – This chapter deals with arms, necks and bust. These movements are not only dramatic in the way they tone and firm the arms and the muscles that support the bust, but are also excellent for correcting posture, getting rid of tension in the neck and shoulders, and realigning the spine.

PART II

The exercises in Part II will take a little longer. Chapters 8 and 9 should not be attempted until you have mastered all the preceding movements and can do them with ease.

Chapter 7 – The Power Stretches will take you about 20–30 minutes and this sequence is fantastic before you go to sleep at night or any time at all when you feel stressed and frazzled. It ends with deep relaxation that will calm both body and mind. It is also great to do after any of the other sequences in this book.

Chapter 8 – is your advanced class. It is most important that you don't even attempt these movements until you feel very comfortable with the preceding chapters. This is a powerful body toning, firming and energizing workout that is fantastic for your shape and flexibility.

Chapter 9 – deals with your yoga hand balances. You may include these, one at a time, when you have gained mastery of the other chapters.

You will find at the end of each chapter in Parts I and II a quick reference chart so that when you have learnt the movements you can see your entire workout on one page.

PART III

In this part, we look at aspects of yoga beyond the exercises.

Chapter 10 – discusses yoga and diet, and emphasizes the importance of selecting foods that will build your health and vitality. There is a chance to try my own personal diet plan which has helped literally thousands of people to their best shape ever.

Chapter 11 – teaches the importance of meditation and how you can use this powerful tool to help keep you relaxed, calm and focused.

Chapter 12 – explores the way in which yoga can help us with many specific health problems, and how it can gradually improve our overall health.

I do hope that by now I have whetted your appetite and you can't wait to get started. Yoga is the most wonderful system for promoting positive health and well-being. Its brilliant combination of amazing exercises, balancing postures, breathing techniques, deep relaxation, meditation and visualization, together with a healthy diet, will help you to radiant health and vitality for many years to come. I hope you come to love it as much as I do.

Enjoy your Yoga!

part one

Your Daily Ten-minute Sequences

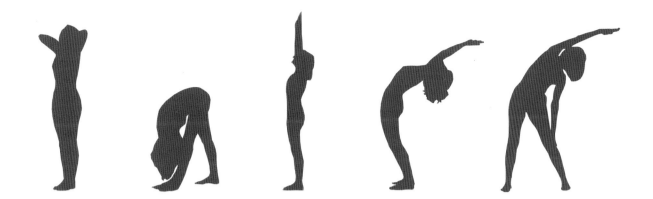

the ten-minute miracle – your morning essential

Have you ever watched an animal wake up after a rest? It stretches its body from top to toe. This gets rid of tension and makes sure it is in perfect condition to start the day. The Ten-minute Miracle is an ideal sequence to start your day. It will greatly improve your shape and flexibility, give you bundles of energy and can be a tremendous help to people with an aching back.

chapter one

1 The Energizing Breath

This is a wonderful breathing exercise. It is a great tonic when done first thing in the morning, but it will give you that 'good to be alive' feeling anytime anywhere.

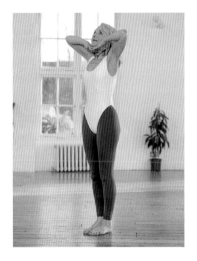

1 Stand straight with your feet together. Place your fingertips interleaved under your chin with your elbows together.

Inhale slowly through your nose for a count of 5. As you do this bring your elbows up as high as possible. Feel the breath at the back of your throat.

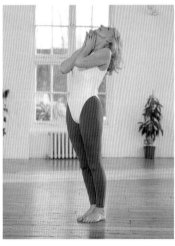

2 Gently let your head drop back and exhale slowly and thoroughly through your mouth. At the end of the exhalation, slowly bring your elbows together as your head slowly returns to its normal position.

Repeat this cycle 5 times to begin with, increasing to 10 times as you become used to the movement.

Note
This movement sounds simple, but standing straight and moving your head back can be quite difficult at first. Please don't worry. Many people have a lot of tension in their necks, but as you progress in yoga you will find it becomes easier. Also, some people feel dizzy or light-headed at first. If so, start by doing the movement only 2 times and take your head just a tiny way back, gradually building up to 5 times as you progress.

Benefits
Because of our sedentary lifestyle, most people use less than one third of their lung capacity. This wonderful movement helps to increase lung capacity, so increasing the oxygen supply to all our cells. This will give you energy and help to relieve stress.

2   Sideways Stretch

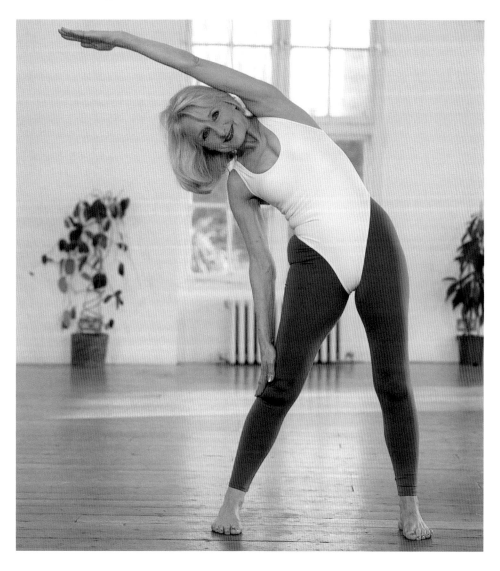

Stand straight with your legs at least 3 feet apart, your toes facing forwards. Inhale deeply and lift your right hand in the air. As you exhale, gently bend over to the left side, sliding your left hand down your left leg. Don't strain. Go just as far as you can with ease.

Breathing normally, hold the position for a count of 5, increasing to 10 as you progress. Inhale and slowly return to an upright position. Exhale, slowly lower your arm and relax. Repeat the movement to the other side, and then repeat the entire movement.

Benefits
This stretch is brilliant for slimming and toning the midriff and waistline, and releasing tension in the lower back.

3   Head to Knee Posture

This is a great stretch for your spine and it also helps to correct imbalances in the lower back.

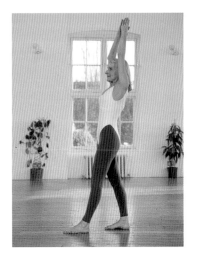

1 Stand straight with your legs together. Inhale and lift your arms up above your head. Place the palms of your hands together and stretch your body upwards. This is great for helping to realign your spine and releasing tension from your entire body.

As you lower your arms, exhale slowly through your nose. Repeat the movement. Now place your right foot about 3 feet in front of your left foot.

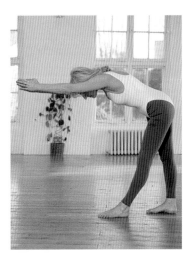

2 Inhale and lift your arms up above your head with your palms together. As you exhale with your head up, back flat and legs straight, start to move forwards aiming your chin just past your knee.

Don't worry if you are nowhere near this position to start with. Just relax in your maximum position and stay there for a count of 5, breathing normally. Take note of your maximum stretch on this side.

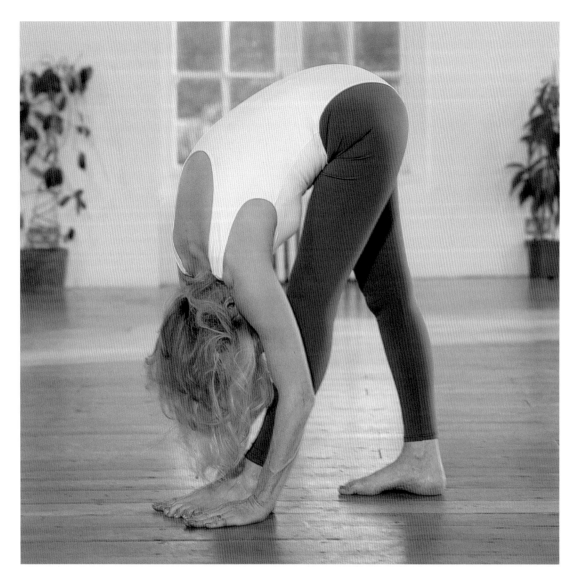

3 Inhale and, lifting your head, slowly return to your upright position. Exhale, lower your arms and relax. Repeat the movement to the other side placing your left foot 3 feet in front of the right. Take note of how far you can manage this side.

Benefits
This movement helps to correct imbalances in the lower back. It firms the backs of the thighs and calves and the bottom, and slims the midriff and waistline.

4   Forwards and Backwards Bend

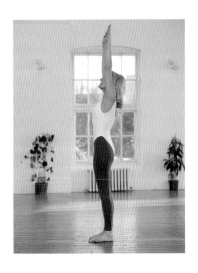

1 Stand straight with your feet about a foot apart, your toes facing forwards. Inhale deeply and slowly lift your arms in the air, stretching them upwards. Exhale slowly through the nose as you move calmly and gently forwards, keeping your back flat and your legs straight.

Relax in your maximum position and stay there, breathing normally. Don't worry if your maximum position isn't very far in the beginning. It will improve quicker than you can imagine. Do not strain yourself.

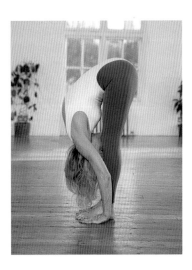

2 Breathing normally, stay in the maximum position for a count of 5, increasing to 10 as you progress. Eventually your chin will be on your shin. Again, this might seem impossible at first, but with practise you'll get there, I promise!

Benefits

An excellent stretch, this gently releases tension from the whole body and ensures wonderful flexibility of the spine. It tones the legs, especially the backs of the thighs, firms the abdomen, midriff, waistline and throat. It is great for the skin and hair because it increases circulation in these areas.

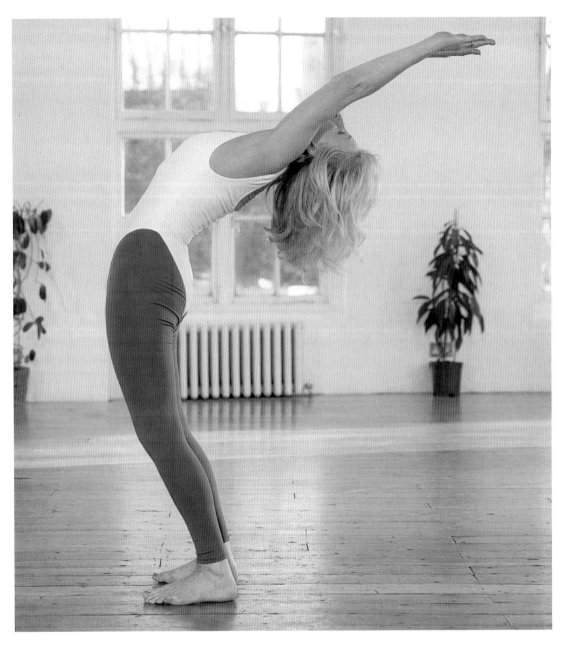

3 Slowly lift your head and, as you inhale, continue to come up slowly into an upright position with your hands stretched up above your head. Keeping your eyes on your thumbs, start to relax gently backwards, exhaling in your maximum position.

Again, don't worry if only an inch is possible to begin with. Breathing normally, hold your backwards stretch for a count of 5. Then inhale and slowly return to an upright position. Exhale, lower your arms and relax. Repeat this movement once.

5 Rishis Posture

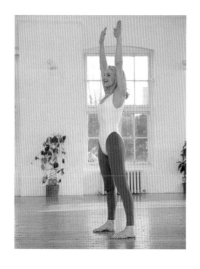

1 Stand straight with your feet 3 feet apart. Inhale and stretch your arms up in the air.

As you exhale, move forwards slowly and, with your legs straight and back flat, grasp your left leg with your right hand. Eventually you will be able to slide your right hand under your left foot, but in the early stages just grasp the leg where it feels comfortable, keeping both legs straight.

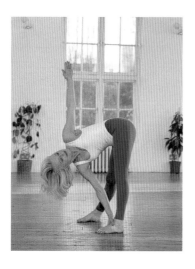

2 Slowly lift your left arm in the air and carefully turn your body so you are looking at your left hand. Breathing normally, hold for a count of 5. Then slowly lower your arm and relax forwards, clasping your legs and gently pulling your upper body towards the legs. Breathe normally.

Inhale and then, as you exhale, grasp your right leg with your left hand and slowly lift your right arm in the air. Again, turn your body carefully to enable you to look up at your right hand. Breathing normally, hold for a count of 5.

Benefits
This is excellent for rebalancing the lower back and is great for people who suffer from tension in this region. I recommend it for tennis players and golfers who can frequently suffer from aches and pain in the lower back. The movement also firms the midriff, waistline, bottom and thighs and keeps the spine in an excellent condition, giving it great flexibility. A real gem of a movement.

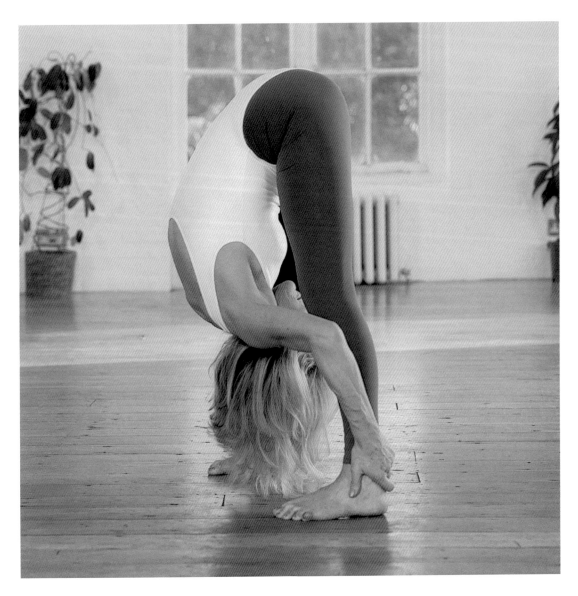

3 Relax forwards, clasping both legs and drawing the body inwards. Inhale and lift your head, then slowly return to an upright position, stretching your arms above your head.

Now place your hands at your waistline with your thumbs in front and fingers behind, and with full lungs gently bend backwards, exhaling as you reach your maximum backwards bend.

Breathing normally, hold your maximum backwards bend for a count of 5. Then inhale as you return to an upright position. Exhale, relax and repeat the entire movement.

6 The Awkward Posture

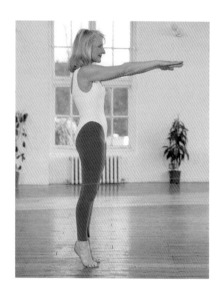

1 Stand straight with your feet about 1 foot apart and your toes facing forwards, not outwards.

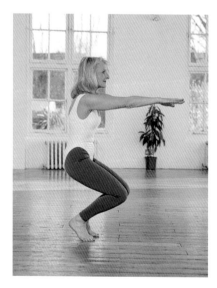

2 Take a deep breath in and, as you exhale keeping your back straight, gently lower your bottom to your heels. Don't worry if only half way is possible in the beginning stages. Just do your best without straining.

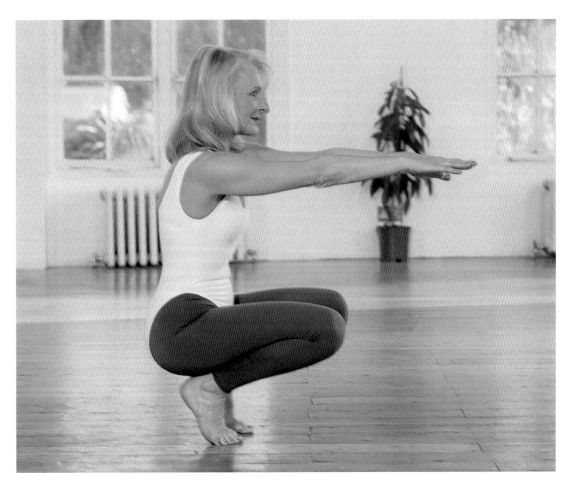

3 Hold your maximum movement for a count of 5. Then inhale and gradually return to an upright position, keeping your back straight (do not bend forwards). Exhale, relax and repeat this movement twice.

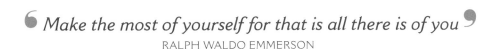

Make the most of yourself for that is all there is of you
RALPH WALDO EMMERSON

Benefits

This does wonders for your thighs – it really tones and firms them. It also greatly improves the flexibility of the knees and strengthens the arches of the feet, and the toes and ankles.

In my opinion, this simple 10-minute sequence is worth its weight in gold. It will give you energy, improve your shape and is excellent for helping with and preventing back problems.

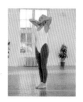 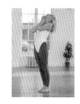 The Energizing Breath

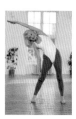 Sideways Stretch

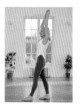 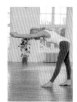 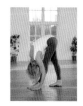 Head to Knee Posture

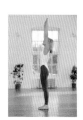 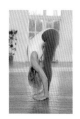 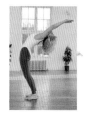 Forwards and Backwards Bend

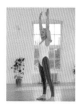 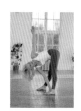 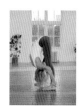 Rishis Posture

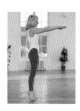 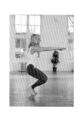 The Awkward Posture

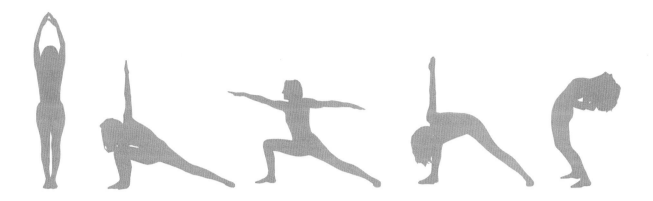

the advanced
ten-minute miracle

Once you feel comfortable with the Ten-minute Miracle and are able to do the movements with ease, then it's good to move on to this stronger stretch. Go carefully.

chapter two

1   Salute to the Sun

This is a wonderful morning stretch, traditionally performed while facing the sunrise. The sun was worshipped in ancient times for its amazing powers. It was thought to be a giver of health and long life.

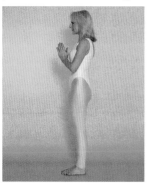

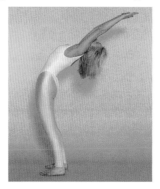

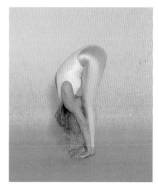

1 Stand straight with your shoulders back, tummy in, hands in prayer and feet together. Beginners may find it more comfortable to have their feet about 1 foot apart. Inhale deeply then exhale slowly.

2 Inhale and lift your arms above your head and, with full lungs, stretch backwards, exhaling in your maximum position.

3 Inhale as you return to a standing position, then exhale as you stretch forwards, aiming your chin to your shins and your hands by your feet. Go as far as you can without strain, aiming to keep your knees straight but, if necessary, bending them to ensure your hands are flat on the floor.

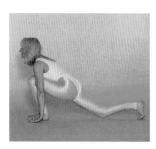

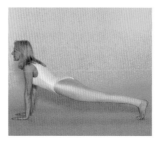

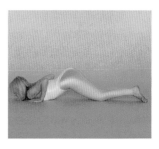

4 Inhale as you stretch your right leg back from the body. Keep the left leg between your hands and look up at the sky.

5 Exhale as you stretch your left leg back.

6 Then lower your entire body to the floor, knees first, then chest, and finally your chin.

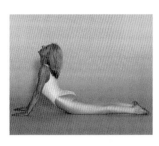 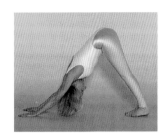 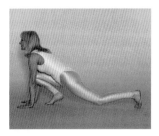

7 With your hands by the side of your shoulders and fingers pointing forwards, inhale as you lift your upper body into the Pose of a Cobra (see page 87), ensuring that your lower abdomen stays on the floor.

8 Tuck your toes under and exhale as you lift your bottom in the air, and stretch your heels to the floor. This is the Pose of a Dog position.

9 Inhale and bring your right foot in between your hands and look up at the sky. Exhale and bring your left foot in and look upwards.

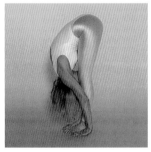 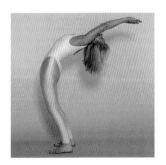 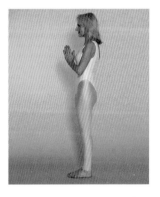

10 Then, with both hands on the floor, gently lift your bottom in the air, aiming your chin to your shins with your hands flat on the floor by your feet.

11 Inhale and slowly lift your head, then your arms. Slowly return to an upright position. Stretch upwards. With full lungs, gently relax backwards, exhaling in your maximum position.

12 Inhale as you gently return to an upright position. Place your hands in prayer, exhale and relax. Repeat the entire routine, this time taking the left leg back first.

Benefits
This is a magical energizing routine. It stretches, tones and firms the muscles in the arms and legs. It trims the midriff and waistline. It gives incredible flexibility to the spine and promotes healthy deep breathing. It really can do wonders for your entire body giving it youthful flexibility and keeping it in great shape.

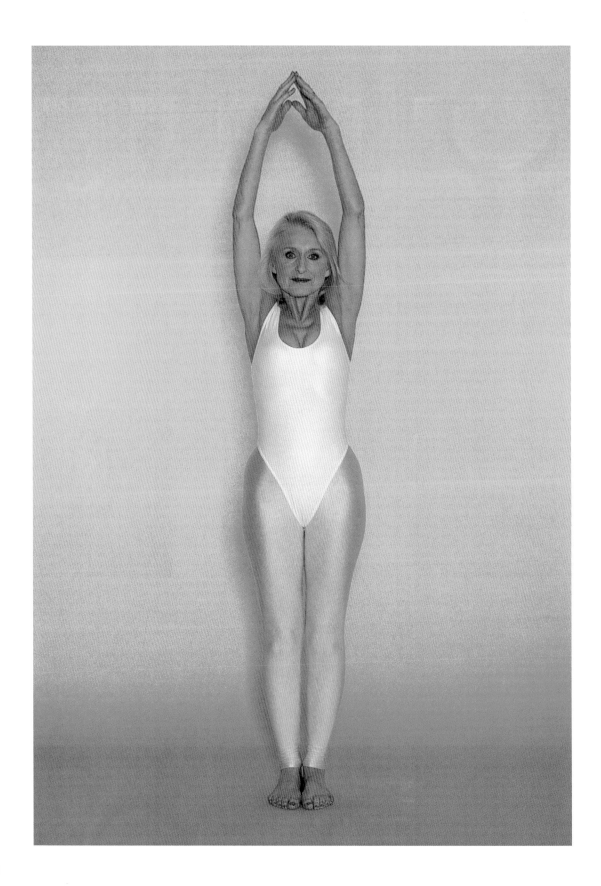

2　The Complete Breath

Stand very straight with your hands by your sides, and your feet about a foot apart. Gently push your abdominals out and slowly inhale through your nose for a count of 5, lifting your arms in the air.

Hold your breath for a count of 5.

Exhale slowly through your nose for a count of 5, lowering your arms as you do so. At the end of your exhalation, gently pull your abdominals in and up without breathing.

This will force the stale air from the base of your lungs. Push your abdominals out and inhale from the base of your lungs. Repeat this breathing exercise 10 times.

As you become more accomplished, gradually increase the inhalation until you are inhaling and exhaling for a count of 10. It will take time to accomplish this and you must never strain the lungs.

Benefits
Yoga teaches us that 'life is breath and he who only half breathes only half lives'. Sadly, most people use only one third of their lung capacity and they breathe much too rapidly. This exercise teaches us to use the whole lung. By pushing the abdominals out, we allow the diaphragm to flatten, and then we gradually fill the lungs from the bottom, aiding extra oxygen absorption by the lungs, so leading to blood rich in oxygen. This is quite difficult to do to begin with, but if you watch small babies breathe while sleeping you will see that this is exactly how they breathe. When people are stressed, they pull their abdominals in during inhalation and push them out as they exhale. This does not allow for adequate oxygen absorption and can lead to low energy levels.

I really recommend that you use this breathing exercise. It will always make you feel calmer, more centred and much more relaxed. It will retrain your lungs and help you to a wonderful feeling of well-being. It can be done in either a standing, seated or lying down position. Obviously, the arm movement is not necessary if you are seated or lying down.

3   The Siamese Posture

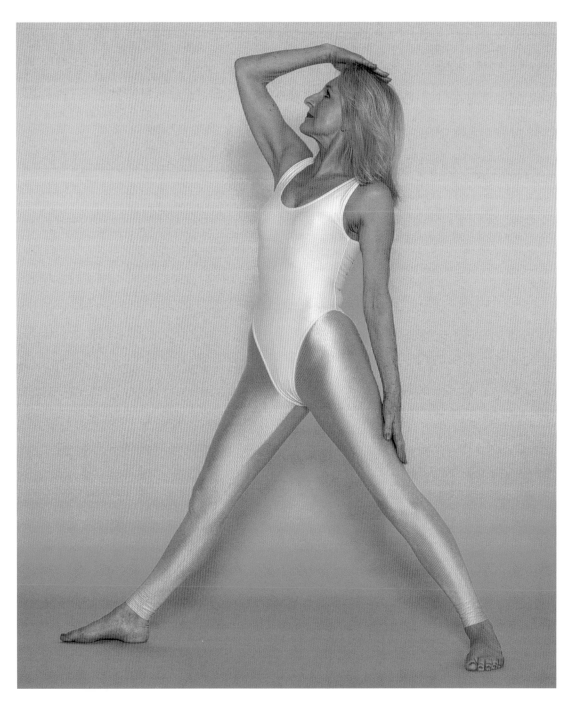

1 Stand straight with your legs about 3 feet apart. Turn your right foot 90° to the right, keeping your left foot facing forwards.

Inhale and place your right hand on the top of your head and look into the centre of your elbow. Keep the left hand on your left thigh.

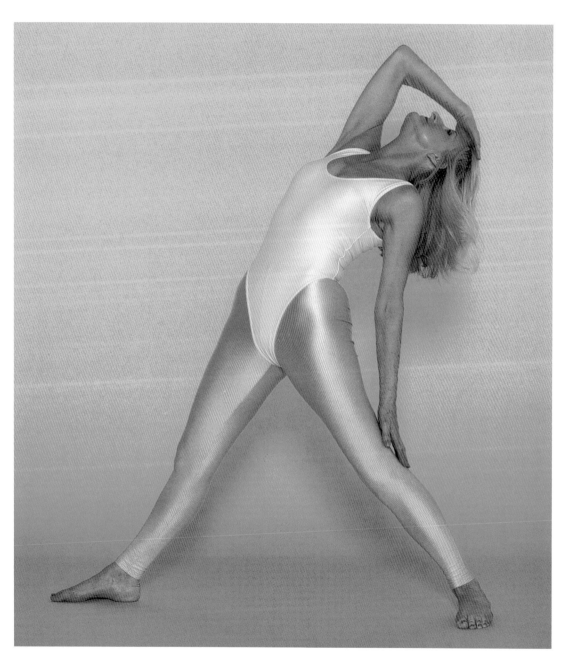

2 As you exhale, slide your left hand down your left leg to your maximum position. Hold for a count of 5.

Inhale slowly and return to an upright position. Exhale and relax and repeat on the other side. Repeat the entire movement.

Benefits
This keeps the spine strong and flexible and really tones the midriff and waistline.

4   The Warrior Posture

Stage one

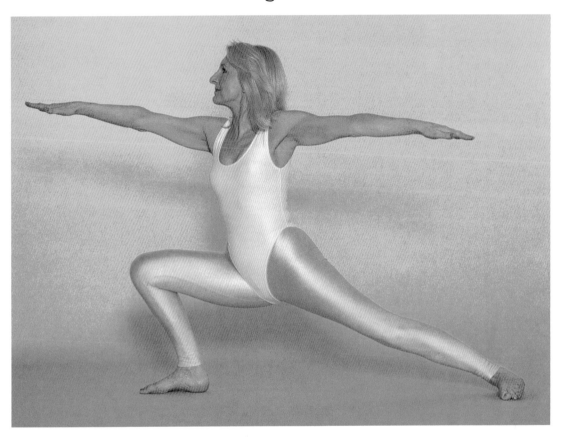

Stand straight with your legs 3–4 feet apart. Turn your right foot 90° to the right and have your arms stretched out to the sides, parallel to the floor at shoulder level. Turn your body so that you are facing over your right hand.

Inhale deeply and, as you exhale, bend your right knee, aiming eventually to have the thigh flat and the left leg straight. Don't worry if this seems impossible to begin with. Do your best without strain.

Breathing normally, hold the position for a count of 5. Inhale as you return to an upright position. Exhale and relax. Repeat the movement on the other side.

Benefits
This movement does wonders for your thighs and buttocks. It streamlines, firms and tones them, and is a great help in removing cellulite. It also streamlines the calves and is excellent for removing tension in the lower back.

Stage two

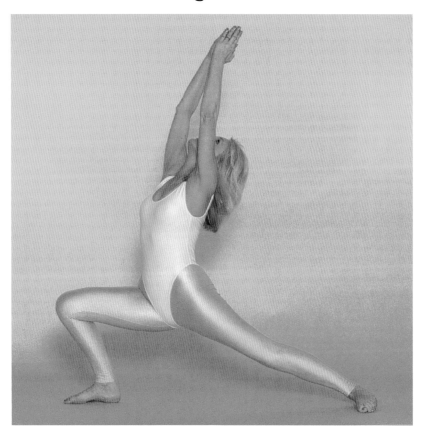

Stand straight with your legs 3–4 feet apart and turn your right foot 90° to the right. Facing towards your right foot, inhale as you lift your arms straight up in the air, placing them together and crossing your thumbs. Relax your head back so you are looking at your hands.

Inhale deeply and, as you exhale, bend your right knee, again aiming to have the thigh flat and the back leg straight. Breathing normally, hold this position for a count of 5.

Inhale as you return to an upright position. Exhale and relax, and repeat to the other side. Repeat the entire movement.

Benefits
This position has the same benefits as Stage one in that it is a terrific toner for the thighs and buttocks, streamlines the legs and releases tension in the lower back. It also firms the jaw and throat.

5   Triangle in Three Stages

Stage one

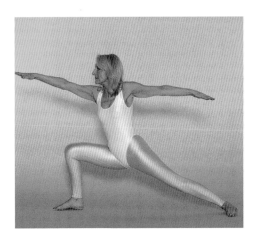

1   Stand straight with your feet 3–4 feet apart. Inhale and turn your right foot 90° to the right, placing your arms out at the sides and parallel to the floor. Turn your body so that you are facing over your right hand.

Exhale and bend your right knee, aiming to have your thigh flat and back leg straight.

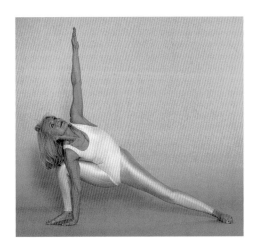

2   Gently lower your right hand to your right foot, aiming to place your hand flat on the floor, and your little finger by your big toe. If this is not possible, clasp the calf in a position that is comfortable for you.

Gently lift your left arm in the air in a straight line with your right foot. Draw your head back in line to enable you to look at the ceiling.

Breathing normally, hold this position for a count of 5, increasing to 10 as you progress. Inhale and return to an upright position. Exhale, relax and then repeat on the left side.

❝ *Infinite energy is at the disposal of man if he knows how to get it, and this is part of the science of yoga.* ❞

ADAMS BECK, *The Story of Philosophy*

Stage two

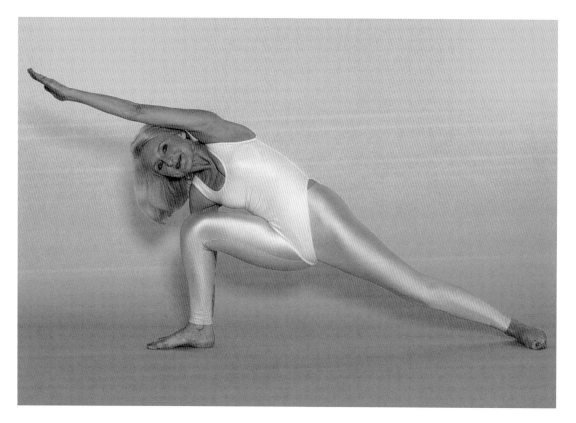

1 Now stand straight with your legs 3–4 feet apart, your arms and feet as in Stage one. Inhale and, as you exhale, bend the right knee, again aiming to have your thigh flat and your back leg straight. Ensure that the outer side of your left foot stays on the floor.

2 Now place your right hand by your right foot, this time with your right thumb by your little toe, with your right knee near your right armpit. If this is not possible just clasp your calf.

3 Draw your left arm alongside your left ear with your arm in a straight line with your left foot and feel that wonderful stretch. Breathing normally, stay in the position for a count of 5, increasing to 10 as you progress. Then inhale as you return to an upright position. Exhale and relax. Repeat to the left side.

Stage three

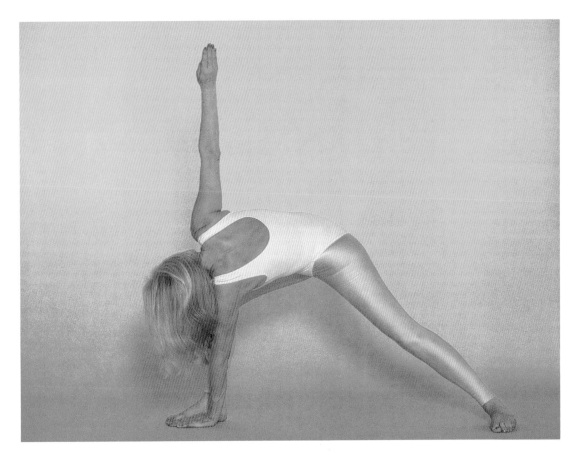

1 Stand straight with your legs 3–4 feet apart and arms parallel to the floor, the right foot at 90° to the right as in Stages one and two. Inhale and, as you exhale, change your arms over so that your left arm is over your right leg.

Inhale and, as you exhale, bend your right knee, aiming to have your thigh flat and your back leg straight. Gently place your left hand flat on the floor with the left thumb by the right big toe or clasp the calf if this is more comfortable for you.

Lift your right arm in the air trying to have it as straight as possible, in line with the right calf. Hold for a count of 5, increasing to 10 as you progress. Inhale and return to an upright position. Exhale and relax. Repeat to the other side.

Benefits
Yes, it is worth it! The triangle works virtually every muscle in your body. It tones, firms and streamlines all the muscles in the arms and legs, and releases tension in the spine. It tones the lower abdominal organs and reduces flab around the midriff and waistline and hips. A real gem!

6 Wide-angled Upward Stretch with Forwards and Backwards Bend

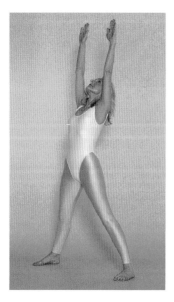

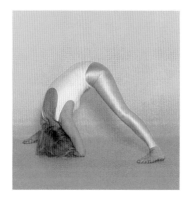

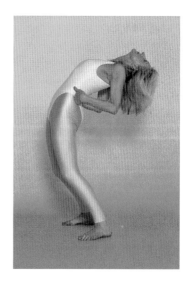

1 Stand straight with your legs 3–4 feet apart and your hands by your sides. Inhale and stretch your arms up in the air.

2 With your back flat and legs straight, exhale slowly as you move into your forwards bend. Breathing normally, relax in your maximum position. Eventually, you will be able to rest your elbows on the floor with your head on your upper arms.

Breathing normally, stay in your maximum position for a count of 5, then slowly lift your head and draw your feet inwards so that they are only about 3 feet apart.

3 Take a deep breath in and return to an upright position with your arms above your head. Place your thumbs in front and fingers behind at your waistline, inhaling deeply.

Bend backwards and exhale in your maximum position. Inhale as you return to an upright position. Exhale, relax and repeat once.

Benefits
This is such a lovely stretch. It stimulates blood flow to the head and neck area, tones the thighs and calves, and slims the midriff and waistline. The backward stretch relieves tightness in the chest and firms the throat and jaw.

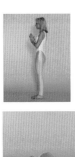

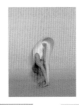
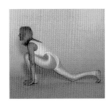
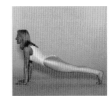

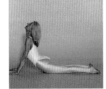
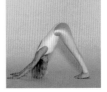
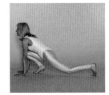

Salute to the Sun

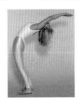
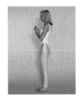

The Complete Breath

The Siamese Posture

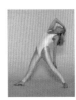

The Warrior Pose (I and II)

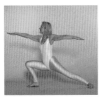
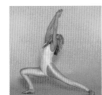

Triangle in Three
Stages

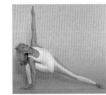
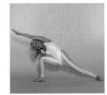
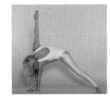

Wide-angled Upward Stretch with
Forwards and Backwards Bend

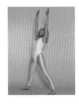

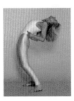

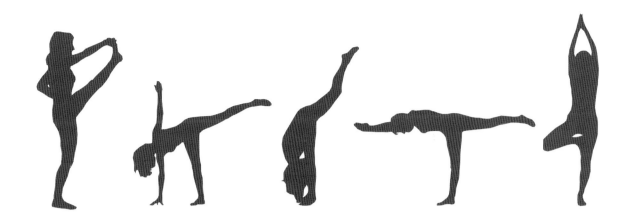

power toning your thighs and bottom

part 1 – yoga balances

Yoga balances firm, tone and strengthen virtually every muscle in the legs and bottom and are excellent for keeping our joints and lower back flexible. They help to strengthen the bones in the legs since the entire weight of the body is transferred to just one leg during these movements.

The balances also teach us the power of focus and concentration as we learn to concentrate on a spot to enable us to do the movements. This takes our mind off our daily activities and gives it a rest, making us concentrate on the present moment.

Although difficult to begin with, most pupils are delighted that they are able to do these movements with ease in a relatively short time.

chapter three

1   Pose of a Tree

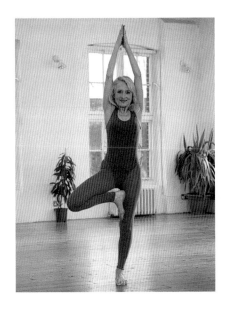

1 Standing straight, inhale and lift your right foot on to your left thigh. This sounds easy but can be quite difficult to start with.

Don't worry or strain yourself. Even if you start by placing your foot on your ankle, calf or knee in the beginning stages, you will assist your joints back to their natural flexibility. Yoga and perseverance will get you there!

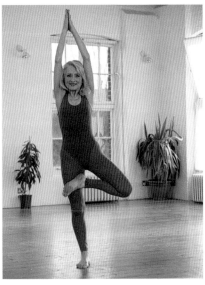

2 Inhale and lift your arms in the air. Placing the palms of your hands together, stare at a spot on the floor or wall to help your balance.

Breathing normally, hold this position for a count of 5, increasing to 10 as you progress. Exhale, lower your arms, replace your foot on the floor and relax. Repeat to the other side, and then repeat the entire sequence.

Benefits
This movement is excellent for toning and firming your inner and outer thighs and strengthening your legs. It also aids the flexibility in your ankles, knees and hips. The balances take your thoughts off your day-to-day activities, so giving your mind a rest.

2 Standing Stick Balance

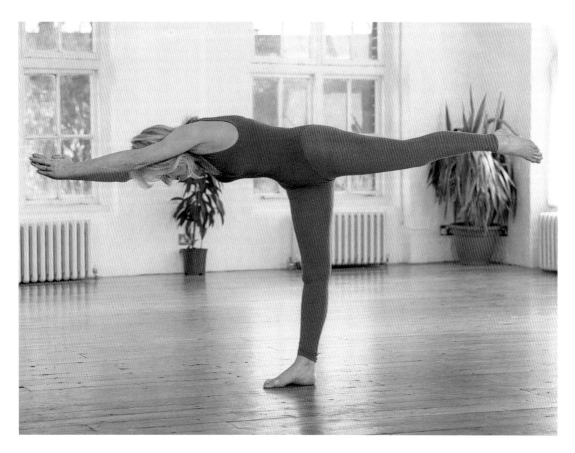

Standing straight with your feet together, inhale and lift your arms in the air, placing the palms of your hands together, crossing the thumbs.

Inhale and place your right foot, 1 foot in front of the left. Exhale and, leaning forwards, lift the left leg so that the entire body resembles a capital T. Stare at a spot to aid your balance. Breathing normally, stretch the body fingers forwards and the left leg back and hold for a count of 5, increasing to 10 as you progress. Inhale and return to an upright position. Exhale and relax.

Repeat on the other side, then repeat the entire sequence.

Benefits
The Standing Stick Balance streamlines the entire body. It firms the hips, thighs and buttocks, strengthens the supporting leg and stimulates the circulation. It is excellent for ridding the body of tension.

3   Half Moon Balance

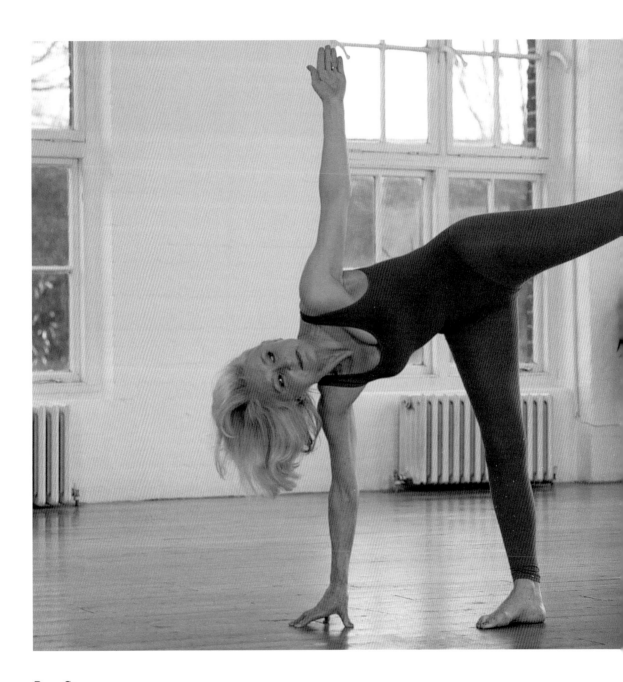

Benefits

This movement tones and slims the hips and thighs, increasing the flexibility in the hips and lower back. It is incredibly good for your balance and coordination.

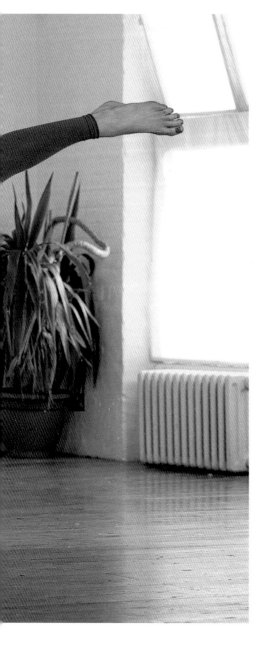

1 Standing straight with both feet together, inhale and stretch your right arm out to the right side, and gently place your hand on the floor. If necessary, bend your knees to enable you to do this.

2 Staring at a spot on the floor, exhale as you lift your left leg in the air. When you have your balance in this position, carefully lift your left arm in a straight line with your right one, and then gently pull your shoulder and head back to gaze at your left hand. Breathing normally, hold for a count of 5, then gradually lower your leg. Inhale and return to an upright position.

3 Exhale, relax and repeat the movement to the other side, then repeat the entire sequence once, increasing the hold to a count of 10 as you progress.

4 Big Toe Balance

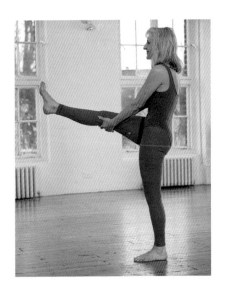

1 Standing straight with both feet together, place your right hand on your right hip. Inhale and take hold of your left big toe in your left hand. Don't worry if this is too difficult at first. Just place both your hands under your left knee.

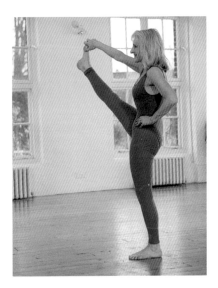

2 Staring at your spot as you exhale, try to straighten your left leg, making sure you keep your right leg perfectly straight. This is difficult at first, but do persevere. It is well worth it. Eventually the leg will straighten.

Hold your maximum stretch for a count of 5 at first, increasing to 10 as you progress. Gently lower your leg to standing position, relax and repeat to the other side. Repeat the entire sequence.

Benefits
This is wonderful for toning and firming the back of your thighs and is a great help in getting rid of cellulite. It also helps your coordination and balance, and releases tension in the hips and lower back.

5   Head to Knee Balance

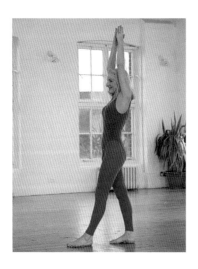

1 With your feet together, lift your arms in the air and place the palms of your hands together, crossing the thumbs. Inhaling, place your right foot about 2 feet in front of your left foot.

As you exhale, carefully stretch forwards aiming your hands to the floor either side of your right foot. In the beginning stages, you may have to bend your right knee to enable you to do this.

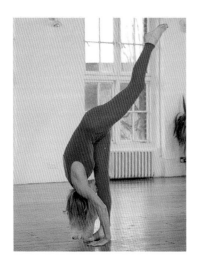

2 Gently lift your left leg in the air, aiming to point the toe towards the ceiling, drawing your chin towards your shin. Relax in the position, breathing normally, and hold for a count of 5. Slowly lower the left leg. Now, with your hands flat on the floor by your right foot, aim to carefully straighten your legs. Don't strain – just persevere!

Inhale as you lift your head, then your arms, and return to an upright position. Stretch your entire body, then exhale and relax. Repeat to the other side and notice if you find one side is easier than the other. This is often the case. Happily, in time yoga will help to correct this imbalance for you.

Repeat the entire movement. Finally, after the last position in your maximum forwards bend, place your feet together and gently aim your chin to just below your knees. Inhale and return to a standing position, stretch your arms above your head. Exhale and relax.

Benefits
This movement tones and firms the thighs and bottom, and helps restore balance and relieve tension in the lower back. It stimulates blood flow to the head and neck area, and helps boost the condition of the skin and hair.

6   Eagle Balance

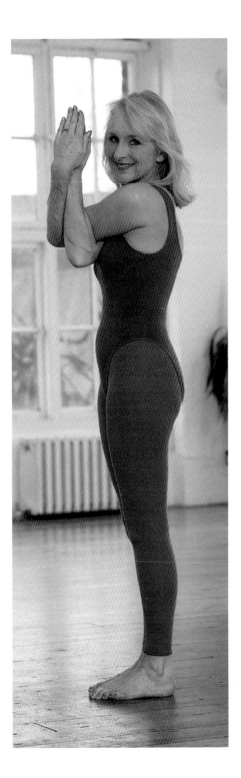

1 Standing up straight with your feet together, stretch both arms straight out in front of you.

Inhale as you cross your right upper arm over your left upper arm, bend the elbows and place both hands in prayer with the thumbs together in line with your nose. Don't worry if your hands do not fit in the beginning. They soon will as flexibility is restored.

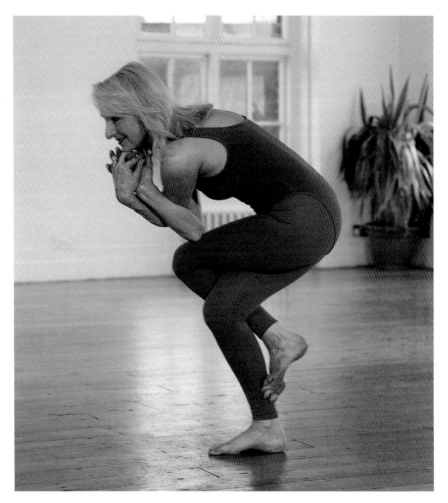

2 Exhale as you repeat this movement with your legs, crossing the right thigh over the left and, bending the left leg, entwine the right foot around the left calf, eventually aiming to have your toes around your calf.

Now interleave your fingers and place your chin on your upper hand, your elbow on your upper knee and hold this amazing balance for a count of 5, breathing normally while staring at a spot on the floor. Inhale as you come out of the position. Stand straight, exhale and relax and repeat on the other side. Repeat the entire movement.

Benefits
This can be a nightmare to start with. It is difficult to balance. Your joints just do not seem to fit together. Your arms won't entwine. Don't worry, we have all started like this – just persevere. Yoga is like an oil can, carefully increasing the flexibility of all your joints in one go. The Eagle Balance tones your upper thighs, helps your concentration and balance, relieves tension in your lower back, and helps stimulate extra blood flow to the lower abdominal organs. None of us realize how quickly our joints can stiffen and this wonderful movement will really help.

7 Dancer's Posture

This is one of yoga's most beautiful movements.

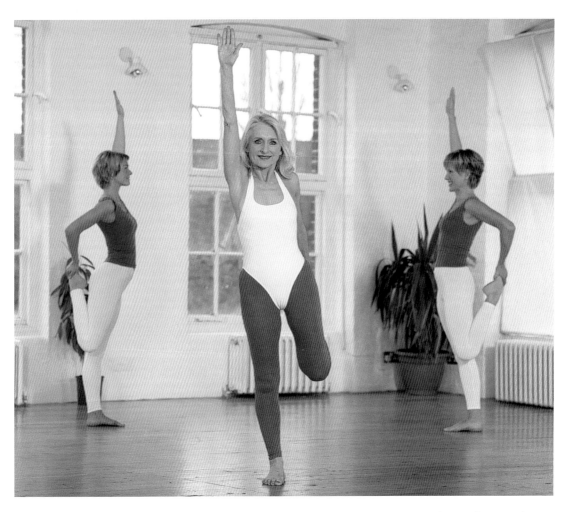

1 With your feet together and with perfect posture, lift your right hand in the air, concentrate on a spot in front of you and inhale.

❝ *Nothing in the world can take the place of persistence. Talent will not, nothing is more common than unsuccessful men with talent. Genius will not, the world is full of educated derelicts. Persistence and determination alone are omnipotent. The slogan 'press on' has solved and always will solve the problems of the human race* ❞

CALVIN COOLIDGE on *Persistence*

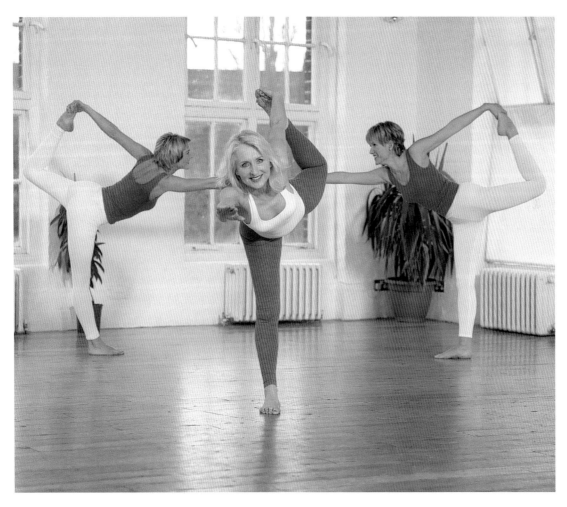

2 As you exhale, grab your left foot in your left hand behind your back, and gently lift the leg as high as possible. Breathing normally, hold for a count of 5.

Gently lower your leg and relax. Repeat to the other side and gradually increase the hold to a count of 10 as you progress. Repeat the entire movement.

Benefits

A beautiful movement, as well as helping your concentration and balance, it relieves tension in your lower back, lifts and firms your bottom, and tones your thighs while strengthening the supporting leg.

39

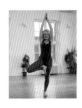 Pose of a Tree

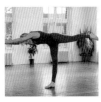 Standing Stick Balance

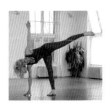 Half Moon Balance

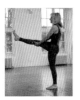 Big Toe Balance

 Head to Knee Balance

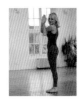 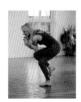 Eagle Balance

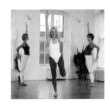 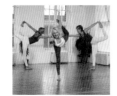 Dancer's Posture

power toning your thighs and bottom

part II – floor movements

chapter four

1 Sideways Leg Raise

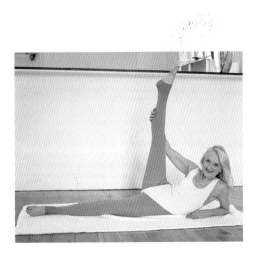

1 Lie on your right side with your body in a straight line, with one leg on top of the other.

Place your lower arm in a supporting position with your fingers pointing in towards your body and your elbow on the floor so that your lower arm supports you.

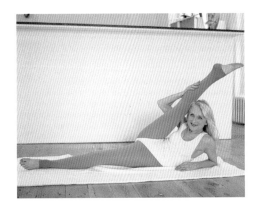

2 Inhale and slowly lift your upper leg to your maximum position without straining. Gently clasp it with your left hand and, keeping the leg straight, aim to draw it gently towards your left ear.

Don't worry if your ear and knee are miles apart at the beginning. This is quite normal and your flexibility will soon improve with practice. Breathing normally, hold for a count of 5 and then gently lower your leg to its starting position. Relax, repeat and then perform the movement twice on the other side.

Benefits
This is an excellent movement for helping your hips to full flexibility. It tones the inner and outer thighs and is a great aid in the removal of cellulite. It can also help to relieve tension in the lower back.

2 Half Locust

Please do not attempt if you are pregnant

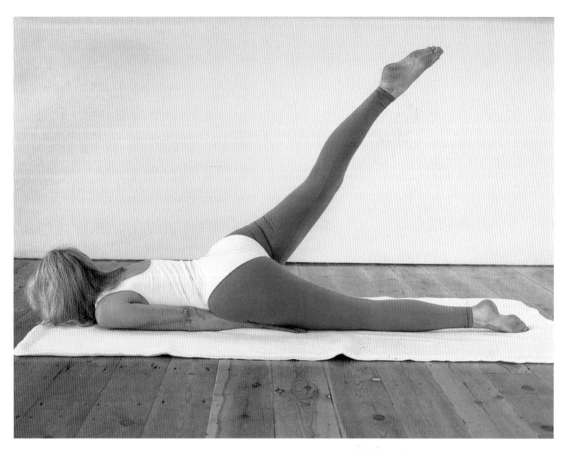

Lie on your stomach with your chin on the floor and your palms facing downwards, under or alongside your thighs.

Inhale deeply and slowly, then as you exhale lift your right leg from the floor, keeping it straight and lifting it as high as you can without strain.

Breathing normally, after holding for a count of 5, gently lower your leg to the floor. Repeat this movement on the other side and then repeat the entire sequence.

Benefits
This movement tones the bottom and thighs, and releases tension in the lower back.

3 Full Locust

Please do not attempt if you are pregnant

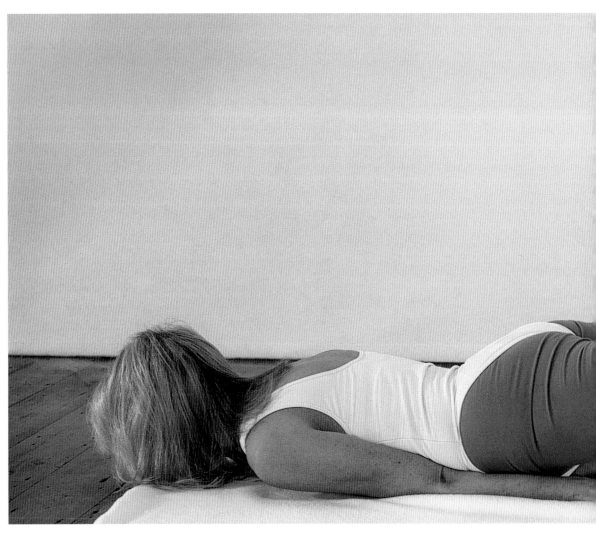

Lying on your stomach with your arms under your body, palms facing downwards, place your chin on the floor, then inhale.

As you exhale, lift both your legs from the floor. Make sure that your upper body remains in a straight line – don't turn or twist – and,

breathing normally, hold the pose for a count of 5.

Gently lower your legs and relax for 20 seconds. Repeat twice.

If you have a weakness in your lower back, wait until the Half Locust becomes really easy before attempting the Full Locust and then only hold for a count of 1, increasing to 5 as you progress.

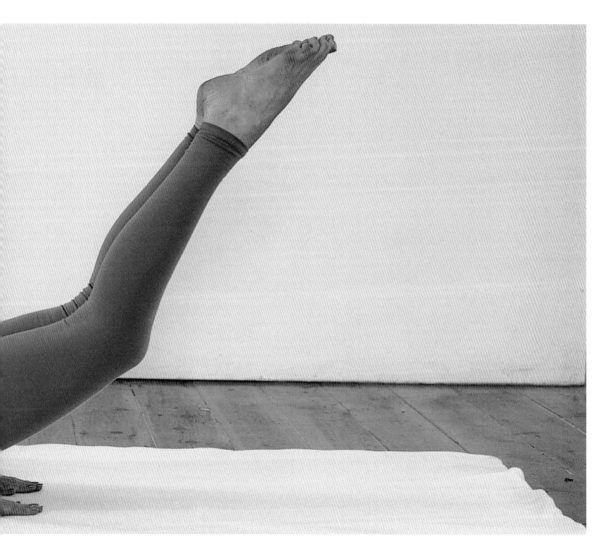

Benefits
This position greatly strengthens the lower back and it can help to relieve constipation and menstrual troubles. It will firm and tone the bottom and thighs and can be a great help in relieving the pain of tennis elbow.

Following the Locust Posture, place your hands either side at shoulder level, then lift your bottom in the air and gently stretch it towards your heels. This is the Pose of a Swan and it is excellent for stretching out, relieving tension and realigning your spine. It is an ideal stretch following the Locust Position.

45

4 Pose of a Monkey

Please do not be put off by the picture of this pose. Yes, it is 'the splits' in ballet, but, no, you are not past it! Daily practice is the key to success in this and every other yoga posture.

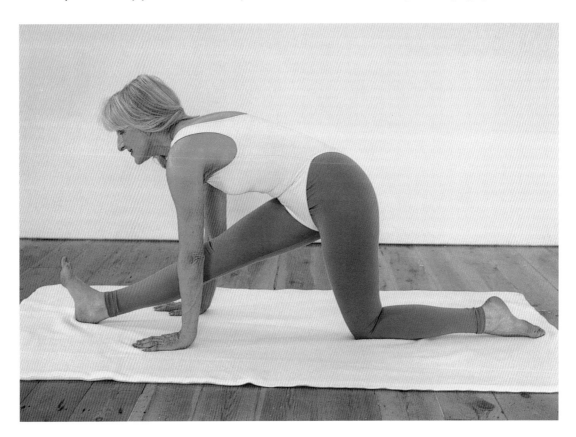

1 Kneel with your knees about 1 foot apart, placing your hands on the floor directly under your shoulders, also about 1 foot apart.

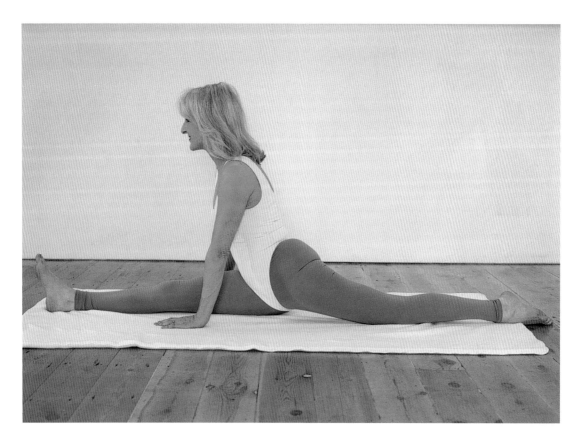

2 Place your right foot in front of you, keeping your weight on your hands. Gently inhale and, with your right heel on the floor, stretch your right leg forwards as you exhale. This may only be a few inches to start with but persevere and you will soon be delighted with the speed of your progress.

Breathing normally and not straining, hold your maximum position for a count of 5, then inhale and return to your 'all fours' position. Exhale and relax. Repeat on the other side, then repeat the entire sequence.

Benefits

This movement looks difficult in the beginning stages, but I have seen miracles happen in this position. You are not too old – I have had pupils start this in their late 70s and manage it. A little daily practice really does make the difference. It is incredibly helpful in relieving lower back pain and sciatica, and is wonderful for toning your thighs and increasing the flexibility of your hamstrings, adductors and quadriceps.

5   Pose of a Heron

Stage one

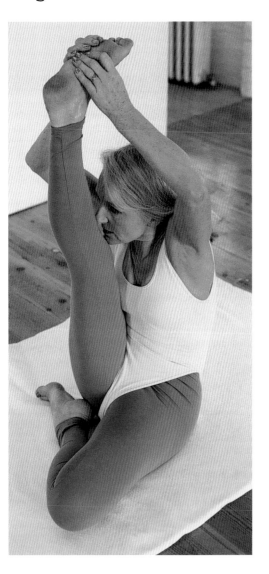

In a sitting position with your legs straight out in front of you, bring your right foot into the space between your legs, placing your heel towards your groin.

Bend your left leg and place your hands under your left foot. Inhale and, as you exhale, aim to straighten your leg without strain. If you cannot straighten it, then place your hands lower down the leg, holding the calf or knee, and then ensure the leg is straight.

With your back and leg straight, and without straining, aim to draw your knee gently to your chin and hold your maximum position for a count of 5. Gently lower the leg, relax and repeat. Repeat the movement twice on the other side. Increase the hold to a count of 10 as you progress.

Benefits
This is a really powerful hamstring stretch. It does wonders for the shape of the back of your thighs and is a great help in getting rid of cellulite.

Stage two is a slightly stronger stretch, so please don't attempt it until you feel comfortable with Stage one.

Stage two

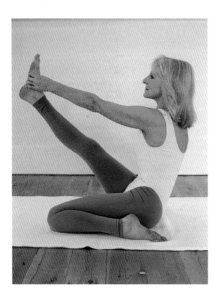

1 Sitting comfortably with both legs straight out in front of you, place your right foot on the outside of the right thigh by your right buttock. Interlock your hands under your left foot and carefully try to straighten your left leg.

If you find it difficult to balance to begin with, place your left hand on the floor to give you support and stretch the left leg, holding it with just the right hand.

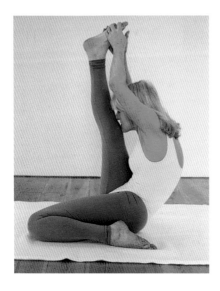

2 Gently draw your left knee towards your chin. Hold your maximum position for a count of 5, gradually increasing to 10 as you progress. Gently lower your leg and repeat, then perform the movement on the other side.

Benefits
This is an incredible toner for your thighs. Yes, it is difficult to do, but persevere. I promise you it is worth it! This movement stretches the hamstrings and smoothes out the back of the thigh while toning and firming the quadriceps on the front of the opposite thigh. It also releases tension in your lower back.

6   Backwards Bend

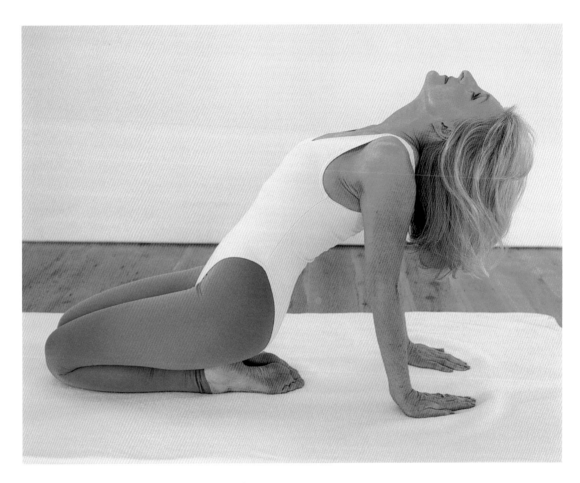

1 Kneel with your bottom on your heels and place your hands on the floor behind you with your fingers pointing backwards.

❝ The secret of making something work in your lives is first of all, the deep desire to make it work, then the faith and belief that it can work; then to hold that clear definite vision in your consciousness and see it working out step by step, without one thought of doubt or disbelief ❞

EILEEN CADDY, *Footprints on the Path*

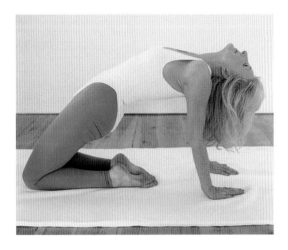

2 Take in a deep breath and gently lift your bottom from your heels. Drop your head back. Exhale in your maximum position and remain in this position for a count of 5.

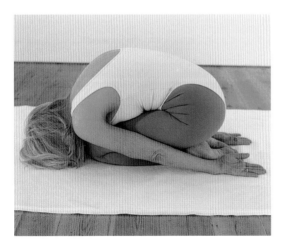

3 Inhaling gently, lower your bottom to your heels. Exhale and place your hands by your side. Relax in this beautiful position, which is called the Pose of a Child. Repeat the movement.

Benefits
The Backwards Bend is one of my favourites. It relieves tension in the chest, firms the neck and throat, corrects poor posture and is wonderful for firming and toning the thighs. It is a great way to stretch out your tensions.

51

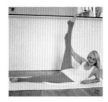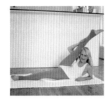 Sideways Leg Raised

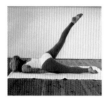 Half Locust

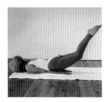 Full Locust

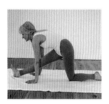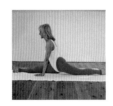 Pose of a Monkey

 Pose of a Heron

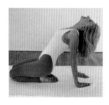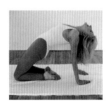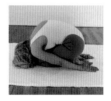 Backwards Bend

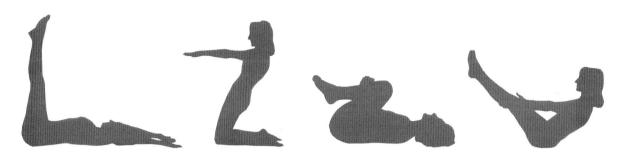

power toning your abdominals, midriff and waistline

chapter five

1 Yoga Abdominal Lift and Contraction

This movement is like a wonderful gift. It only takes 30 seconds a day and is brilliant for those stomach muscles! It must be done on an empty stomach – the ideal time to do it is before breakfast.

Please do not attempt if you are pregnant

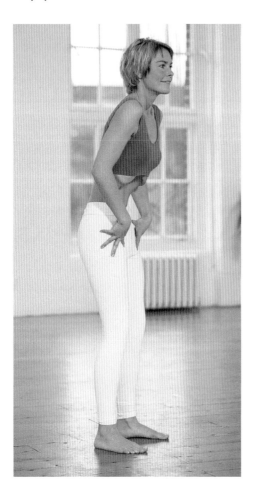

Don't worry if you do not appear to be getting much movement in the beginning stages – just persevere. The resulting slimmer, firmer and flatter tummy is well worth it!

Stand straight with your legs about 1 foot apart, placing your hands on your upper thighs.

Inhale deeply, then exhale fully. Keeping the air out of your lungs pull your abdominals in and up. Hold for a count of 10, then release the abdominals, inhale and relax. Repeat the movement twice.

You can then try an abdominal contraction. Inhale, then exhale and lean slightly forwards. Keeping all the air out of your lungs, snap your abdomen in and out 10 times, increasing gradually to 20 as you progress. Relax, inhale and repeat the movement twice.

Benefits

The abdominals drop as we get older and this movement is invaluable for keeping the abdomen firm, toned, uplifted and youthful.

The contraction massages your internal organs (your small intestine, colon, pancreas, gall bladder and heart). The movement can help tremendously in stimulating peristalsis and relieving constipation and gives relief to those who suffer from irritable bowel syndrome and abdominal bloating.

We do not always appreciate how much our body is affected by our mind. We all have experienced a 'gut reaction', the feeling of a knot in the lower abdomen. This wonderful movement is excellent for helping to release this feeling of tightness.

2 Tummy and Thigh Toner

This deceptively simple movement is like dynamite!

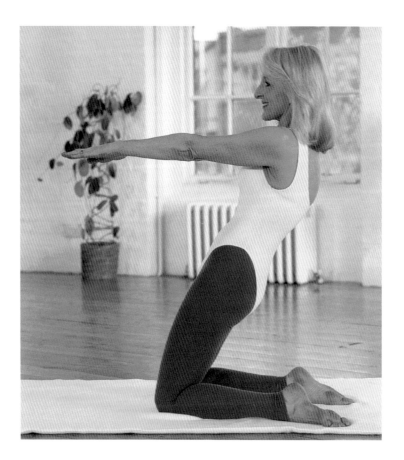

Kneel with your knees about a foot apart.

Lift your bottom from your heels and, keeping your back straight, place your arms parallel to the floor making sure that your thighs are straight and perpendicular to the floor.

Inhale and, as you exhale, lean back a small way, increasing the stretch as you progress. Don't let your bottom sag. Breathing normally, hold the position for a count of 5, then inhale and return to an upright position. Repeat the movement twice.

Benefits

This powerful movement really tones and firms your tummy. It gives your thighs that beautiful firm, toned, slim yoga shape.

3   Pose of a Boat

Please do not attempt if you are pregnant

This is a fantastic firmer for both tummies and thighs. It also greatly strengthens the lower back. Sit on a thick mat or blanket for this exercise.

Stage one

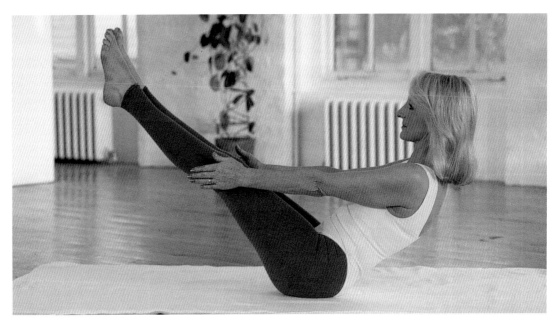

Sit straight with both legs straight out in front of you.

Stretch out your arms parallel to the floor. Inhale and, as you exhale gently, lift your legs from the floor and balance on your bottom. Hold the position for a count of 1 to begin with, gradually increasing to 10 as you progress, then gently lower your legs to the floor and relax.

Repeat the movement twice. This can be hard work but move carefully and build it up gently. Remember, never strain in the posture.
Following the movement, lie on your back, draw your knees to your chest and gently rock your back from side to side to relieve any tension in your lower back.

Stage two

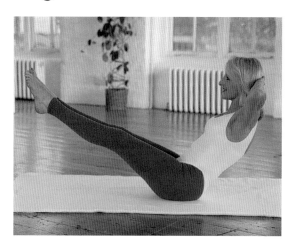

Sitting on your mat with both legs stretched out in front of you, place your hands interlocked behind your head.

Take a deep breath and, as you exhale gently, lift your legs from the floor. Hold for a count of 1 to start with, increasing to 10 as you progress. This is very powerful – do not strain!

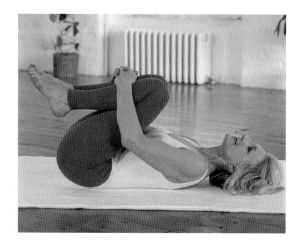

Gently lower your legs to the floor and then relax. Repeat the movement twice.

Following the movement, lie down and gently draw your knees to your chest and rock from side to side.

Benefits
Again, this is a powerful toner for your abdomen, thighs and lower back.

4　Slow Motion Firming

Please do not attempt if you are pregnant

This beautiful sequence not only gives you a lovely firm, strong and flat tummy, but also is delightfully relaxing and is great to do after a long hard day before going to sleep at night. The movement is performed in one slow continuous motion.

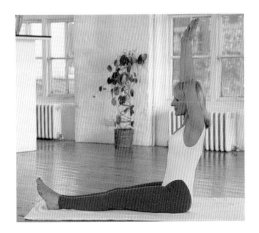

1 Sit up with your back straight and with both legs straight out in front of you and together. Place both arms parallel to your legs. Inhale and lift your arms in the air.

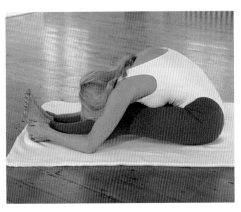

2 Exhale as you slowly move forwards, keeping your back and legs straight, do not strain, just allow your body to flow easily and gently into your maximum position. You should eventually aim to clasp your feet and draw your chin to your knees.

> *To the dull mind all nature is leaden. To the illuminated mind the whole world burns and sparkles with light.*
>
> RALPH WALDO EMMERSON

Benefits
This beautiful sequence will deliver the results you want – a beautiful, firm tummy and nice strong back – and it will really relax you. If your back is stiff and tense, you may toss and turn and find sleep difficult. This movement is perfect for unwinding this tension and helping you to deep restful sleep.

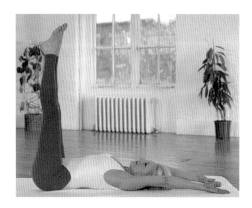

3 Inhale as you slowly return to an upright position, then exhale as you gently lie flat. Place your arms flat on the floor behind your head. Inhale and gently bend your knees, lift your legs up and straighten them so that they are at right angles to your body.

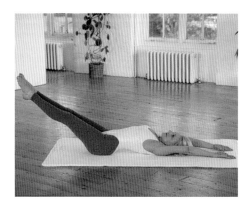

4 Exhale as you slowly lower your legs to the floor. In the beginning stages, make this part of the movement relatively fast, then slow it down as your abdominals firm and strengthen.

For people with weak backs, you may feel a small pull in your lower back to start with. If this occurs, immediately bend your knees and then continue to lower your legs with your knees bent. As you progress you will find that you will be able to go further before having to bend your knees.

Inhale as you slowly come up into a sitting position, stretching your arms up in the air. If you find this difficult in the beginning stages, then use your elbows to help you push off. Exhale as you relax and stretch forwards into a back stretch.

Repeat this sequence twice, increasing to 4 times as your back and abdominals become stronger. Then lie down, draw your knees into your chest and gently relax your back into the floor, gently rocking from side to side. Then lie flat, slow your breathing down, and relax.

Well done!

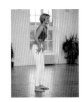 Yoga Abdominal Lift and
Contraction

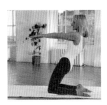 Tummy and Thigh Toner

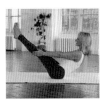 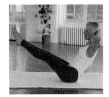 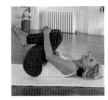 Pose of a Boat

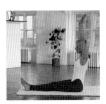 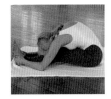

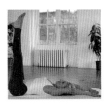 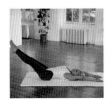 Slow Motion Firming

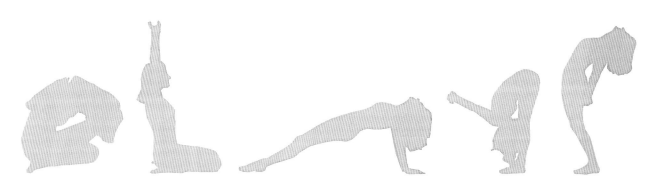

power toning your arms, bust and neck

chapter six

1　The Chest Expansion

These movements are not only dramatic in the way that they tone and firm the arms and the muscles that support the bust, but they are also excellent for correcting posture, relieving tension in the neck and shoulders, and realigning the spine.

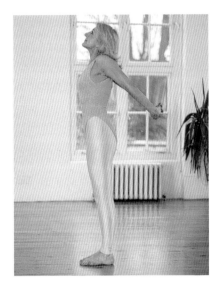

1 Stand with your feet together and your back straight. Interlock your hands behind your back, gently pulling your shoulders back and straightening your arms.

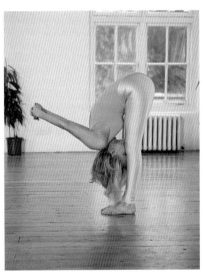

2 Inhale and lift your arms up as high as possible behind your back, then exhale as you slowly bend forward into your maximum forward bend, keeping your back and legs straight. Breathing normally, relax and hold your maximum position for a count of 5.

Your aim is to be able to place your chin on the top of the shin, just under the knee. It will happen eventually, but remember not to strain!

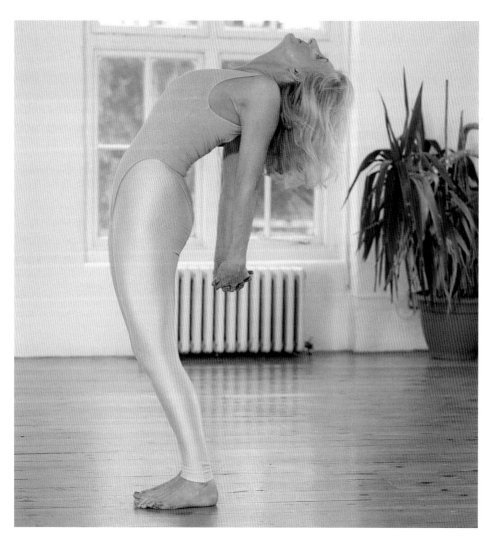

3 Inhale and lift your head, then slowly return to an upright position and gently bend backwards, pulling your arms back down and under your bottom. In your maximum position, exhale, and hold for a count of 5.

Inhale and return to an upright position, hold your arms up behind your back for an extra count of 2, then lower them and relax. Repeat the movement twice.

Benefits

On the physical level, this movement is amazing in how it tones your upper arms and releases the tension in the back of your neck and shoulders. In the forward bend it tones the back of your thighs and calves and stimulates blood flow to the head and neck area, so benefiting your skin, hair and brain cells. While bending backwards, the movement frees the chest of tension and firms the jaw and throat.

The tensions of the mind are frequently stored in the back of the neck (the proverbial pain in the neck) and lumbar spine. This powerful movement carefully relaxes both these areas.

2   Pose of a Plane

This movement, as well as strengthening your arms and shoulders, releases tension in the lower back.

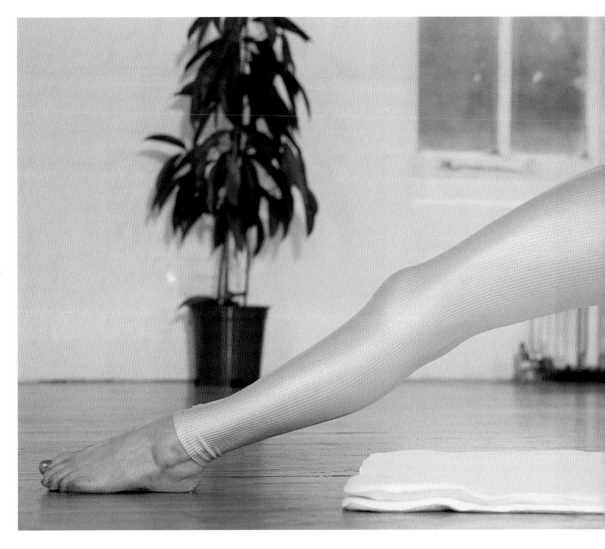

The year's at the spring, And the day's at the morn;
Morning's at seven; The hill-side's dew-pearled;
The lark's on the wing; The snail's on the thorn;
God's in His heaven, All's right with the world!
ROBERT BROWNING, from 'Pippa Passes'

Sit straight with your hands comfortably on the floor behind you, about 1 foot behind your bottom with your fingertips facing backwards. Your legs should be straight out in front of you.

Inhale and, as you exhale, keeping your body in a straight line, place your weight on your arms and gently lift your body from the floor. Ensure that your legs are straight and your toes are on the floor. Hold for a count of 1 at first, increasing to 10 as you become stronger.

Slowly lower your bottom to the floor and relax. Repeat this movement once.

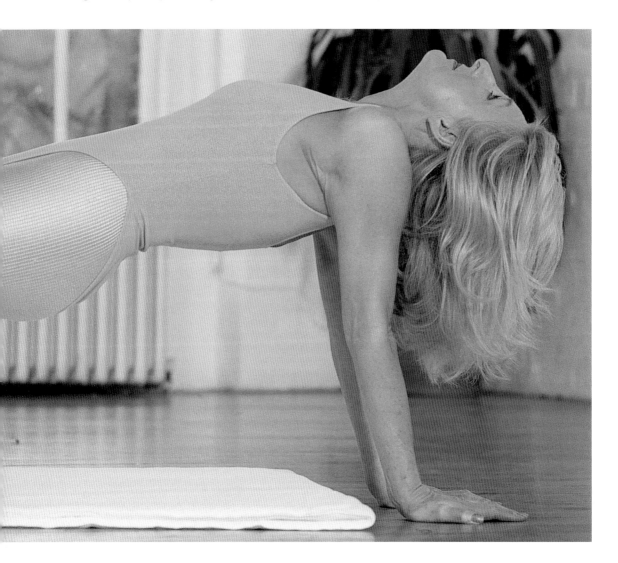

Benefits
This is so good for the strength of your hands, arms, wrists and fingers. It gives great shape to your upper arms and shoulders. It helps to correct drooping shoulders and releases tension in the lower back.

3   Sideways Body Raise

This is another excellent arm shaper and strengthener. We have a built-in response to put a hand out to break a fall should we slip. If our wrists and arms are weak, this can easily result in a break. Yoga hand balances such as this perfectly address the problem. If you have had a wrist or arm problem, follow the directions below but do not lift your bottom – just put a little weight on your hands to strengthen them gradually. Follow these instructions only when your arms are sufficiently strong.

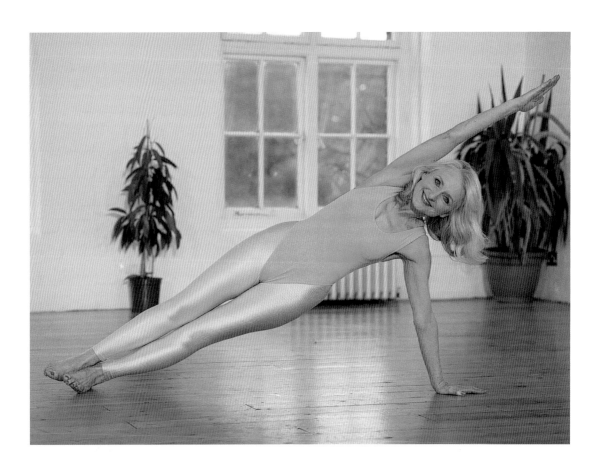

Place both hands on the floor to the right-hand side of your body. Keep your knees bent and make sure that your hands and feet are on a non-slip surface. Inhale and as you exhale, lift your body from the floor, ensuring that your weight is supported on both hands and both feet.

Adjust your body so that your right shoulder is directly above your right wrist and that your arm is straight. Lift your bottom and make sure the left foot is on top of the right one and that the body is in a straight line.

When, and only when, you feel strong enough, lift your left arm from the floor and stretch it in a straight line, with the inside of the arm alongside your left ear. Concentrate on a spot on the floor and hold your balance for a count of 5, then relax. Gently lower your bottom to the floor and repeat on the other side. Repeat the whole movement once.

Benefits
An excellent arm toner and firmer that gives excellent shape to your upper arms and shoulders. This movement greatly strengthens the wrists, hands, elbows and shoulders. An extra benefit is in the way it stretches the hands. For those who spend many hours at the computer, the wrists can become very stiff and painful and this movement can help tremendously.

4   The Mountain Pose

We tend to 'shoulder our problems' and this beautiful movement helps lift away the pressures of the day. Although yoga cannot remove the problem, it can help remove the tension resulting from the problem.

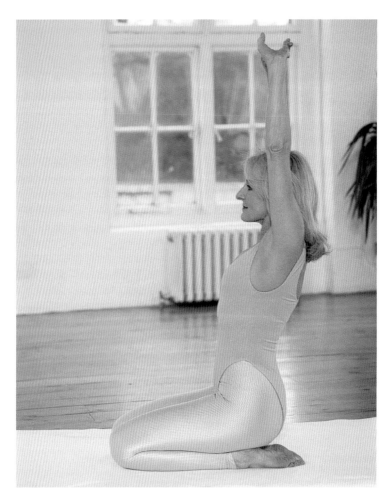

1 Kneel down on your mat with your bottom on your heels. Some people find this very difficult to begin with. You can help yourself by placing a thick cushion on top of your calves under your bottom. If this still doesn't feel comfortable, then sit in a cross-legged position.

Interlock your hands in front of you so that you are looking into the palms, then gently turn them inside out so that you are now looking at the back of your hands.

Inhale and stretch your arms up above your head. Exhale and straighten your arms – imagine you are pushing the ceiling a little higher. Breathing normally, hold this stretch for a count of 5 in the maximum position. Inhale, undo your hands, exhale and slowly lower them. Repeat the movement.

Advanced Mountain Pose

Once your knees have acquired sufficient flexibility to do the Mountain Stretch with ease, then (and only then) try this slightly stronger stretch.

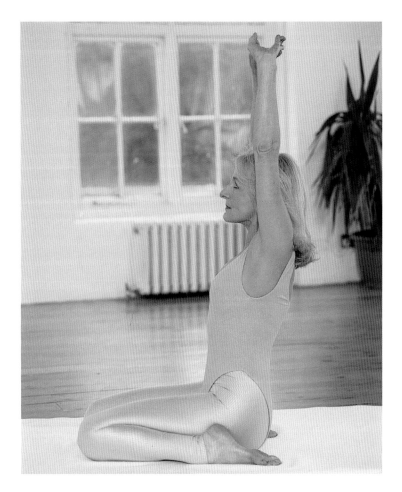

2 With your knees a hip width apart, place your hands on the floor and, keeping your weight on your hands, aim to lower your bottom between your heels.

Once you can sit comfortably in this position without strain, repeat the Mountain Posture for this advanced stretch – inhale, interlock your hands, turn them inside out, exhale, push them upwards aiming to straighten the arms. Breathing normally, hold for a count of 5, then exhale and relax. Repeat twice.

Benefits
The Mountain Posture helps to lift the pressures of life from your shoulders, it tones and firms your upper arms and enhances the flexibility of your wrists and fingers. It is excellent for strengthening the spine and, in the advanced stage, ensures flexibility of the hips, knees and ankles.

5   Pose of a Cow

This position helps to correct neck tension and realign the neck and shoulders. These can frequently be imbalanced due to such things as carrying heavy shoulder bags, constant use of one arm at the expense of the other and playing lop-sided sports.

This position can be astounding, with one side seeming easy and the other almost impossible. It is good to discover our imbalances. Rest assured that daily practise of this movement will gradually help correct the problem for you. Repeat the entire sequence just once.

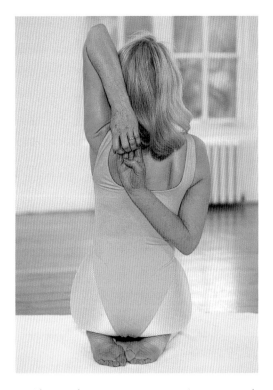

1 Sit in a kneeling position with your bottom on your heels. If this is not possible, adopt a cross-legged pose.

Inhale, lift your right hand in the air and drop it over your right shoulder. Exhale and lift your left arm up behind your back, aiming to join your hands in a clasped position. Don't worry if you cannot join them at first, just practise and soon you will be able to. In the meantime, remember your maximum position is fine.

Inhale and, as you gently exhale, bend forwards and aim your forehead to the floor. Breathing normally, hold this position for a count of 5, then inhale and return to an upright position. Unclasp your hands, relax and then repeat on the other side, noticing if there is a difference between the two sides.

Advanced Pose of a Cow

Once you find the Pose of a Cow easy in all respects, you can try the advanced stage for a stronger stretch. Before you attempt this you must be able to sit on your heels with ease.

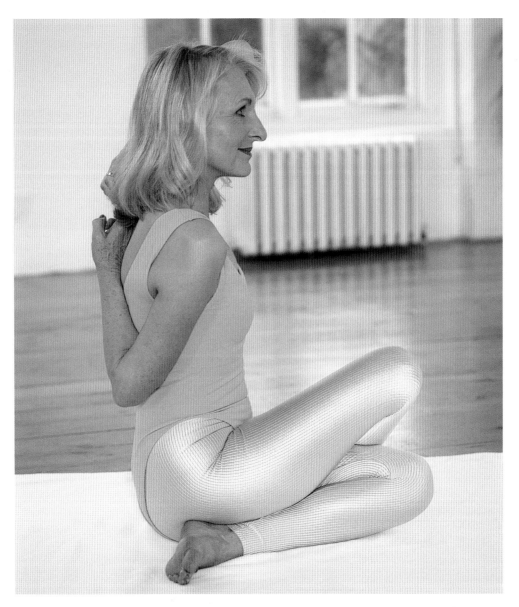

2 In an all fours position, ensuring that your weight is on your hands, place your right leg over your left and then gently lower yourself down to sit between your heels. Go carefully. It may take a while to accomplish this position and remember that the only way to get there is daily practise without strain. If it is too difficult, just remain in a kneeling position. Lift your right arm in the air and drop it down behind your right shoulder. Take the left arm up behind your back and clasp your hands together.

71

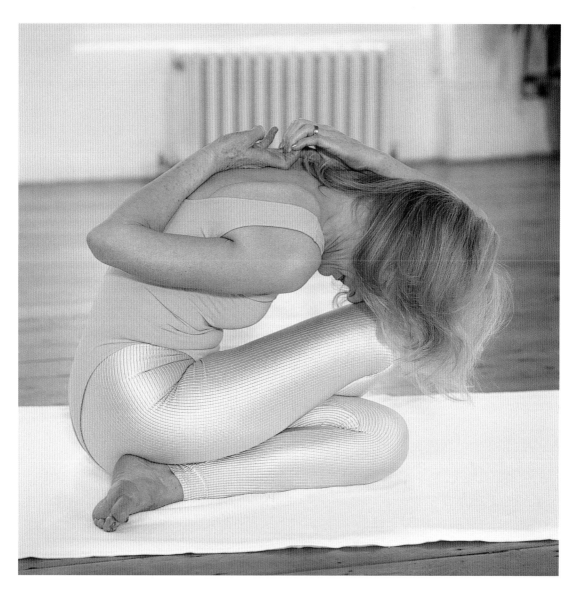

3 Inhale and, as you exhale gently, bend
forwards and place your forehead on your
upper knee. Breathing normally, stay in this
position for a count of 5, then inhale and
return to an upright position. Exhale and relax
and perform the movement on the other side.
Repeat the movement once on each side.

Benefits
*Pose of a Cow helps to correct imbalances in your shoulders. It tones and firms your upper
arms and firms the muscles that support the bust. In the advanced position, it is excellent
for toning the thighs and ensuring the flexibility of your hips, knees and ankles.*

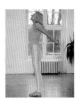 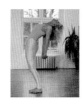 The Chest Expansion

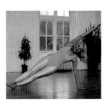 Pose of a Plane

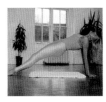 Sideways Body Raise

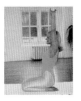 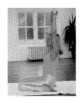 The Mountain Pose and
Advanced Mountain Pose

 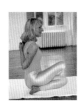 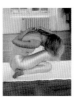 Pose of a Cow and
Advanced Pose of a Cow

part two

More Amazing Movements

power stretching

Yoga's beautiful stretches reshape the entire body and help us unwind, relax and refocus. This particular workout can be done any time but is especially helpful to relax and soothe you before sleep.

chapter seven

1   Alternate Leg Pull

This is a fantastic aid to flexibility in the hips, knees and ankles. It is also calming and relaxing.

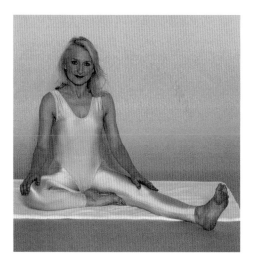

1 Sit straight with both legs straight out in front of you.

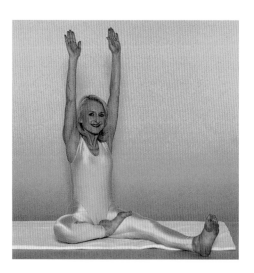

2 Lift your right foot onto your left thigh and place your right hand on your right knee. Now gently bounce your right knee 6 times towards the floor. Don't worry if your joints are really stiff to start with. This is quite normal.

Now, keep your foot on your left upper thigh if it is comfortable and the knee is able to rest easily on the floor. If this is not possible – and it rarely is to start with – then place the right heel on the floor near your groin. Inhale deeply and lift both your arms in the air.

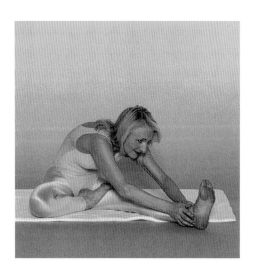

3 Exhale and reach forwards, keeping your back and left leg straight. Try to clasp your left foot in both hands. Aim your chin toward your shin and your chest to your upper thigh. Don't worry if this feels impossible to start with.

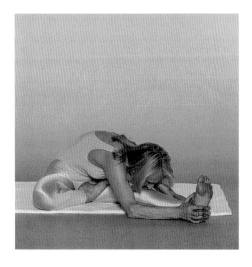

4 Breathing normally, relax in your maximum position, holding for a count of 5. Inhale and then slowly return to a sitting position. Exhale, relax and gently massage your ankles and knees in a slow circular motion to encourage flexibility in your joints. Do the movement twice on each side.

Benefits
This movement will quickly relieve stiffness in your ankles, knees and hips. It also removes tension from your lower back and is a great help in restoring the balance of your lower back and hips. (It is so easy to become lop-sided due to poor posture or imbalanced sports activities.) The movement stimulates blood flow to the abdominal organs and tones your hamstrings and calf muscles.

77

2   Thigh Stretch

This is great for increasing the flexibility of your hips and is a boon during pregnancy.

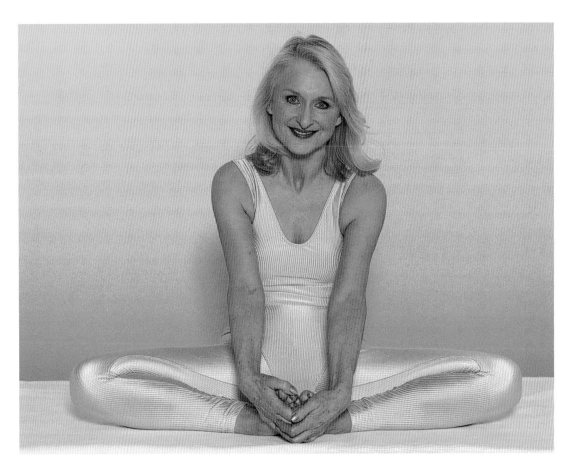

Sit straight with the soles of your feel together near to your groin. Clasp your hands around your feet and take a deep breath in and, as you exhale, gently aim your knees to the floor. Don't be discouraged if they do not move much at first. Just practise and you will see the results sooner than you expect.

Breathing normally, hold your maximum position for a count of 5, then slowly inhale as your knees return to an upright position. Exhale and relax. Repeat the movement 5 times.

Benefits
With our sedentary life, it is easy to allow our joints to become stiff – 'If you don't use it you lose it'. This movement will keep your hip joints flexible and, if you are pregnant, flexible hips will really help with your baby's delivery. It is also fantastic in the way it tones your inner thighs.

3 Pose of a Star

This position relieves tension in your lower back, and tones and firms your inner and outer thighs.

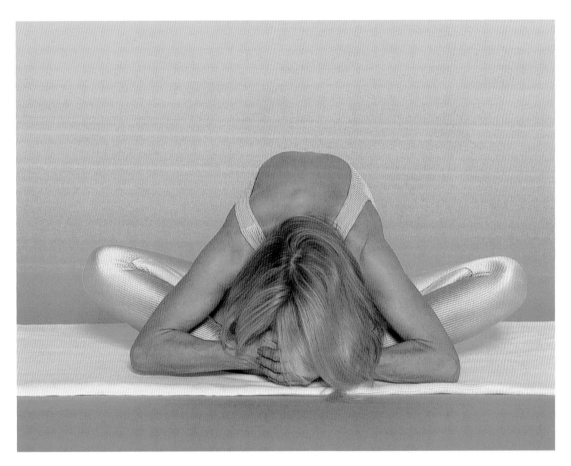

Sit straight with your hands clasped around the sides of your feet and draw your feet in towards your groin as in the Thigh Stretch.

Inhale deeply and, as you exhale, gently open your thighs, pressing your knees as far outwards as they can go and then bend your elbows. Keep your back straight, and gently stretch your chin towards your toes. Breathing normally, hold your maximum position for a count of 5. Inhale and slowly return to an upright position. Exhale and relax. Repeat the movement twice.

Benefits
This movement is excellent for increasing the flexibility of your hips. It tones your inner and outer thighs, releases tension in your lower back and is very beneficial for the health and tone of your pelvic floor.

4 The Lotus Positions

Once you have increased the flexibility of your hips, knees and thighs by the previous three movements, it is then time to try the Lotus Positions.

The Half Lotus

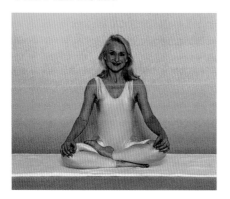

Sit straight with both your legs straight out in front of you and bring your right heel against your groin. Inhale and then gently try to lift your left foot onto your right thigh. Don't worry if you cannot do this yet.

Breathing slowly and deeply, stay in this position for a count of 10, then gently unwind your legs, stretch them out and try the movement with your right foot on your left thigh. Note that in the beginning stages, one side is often easier than the other.

The Full Lotus

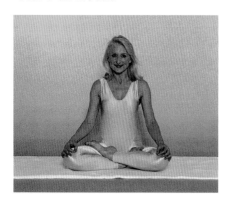

Sit up straight with both legs out in front of you. Gently aim to lift your right foot onto your left thigh, then carefully lift your left foot onto your right thigh. It may be a little while before your joints are sufficiently flexible to achieve this. Don't strain!

Once you are able to hold the position, then stay in it for a count of 10, breathing calmly, slowly and deeply. Then gently come out of it.

Repeat, this time placing your left foot on to your right thigh and then your right foot on to your left thigh. It is important that you alternate your legs in this posture to ensure even and correct development of your flexibility.

Benefits
I have to admit it. This pose is seldom comfortable to start with. But once your joints are sufficiently flexible for you to do it with ease, it is really relaxing – honestly! It is recommended for breathing exercises and meditation, because the spine is erect and the legs entwined so that fidgeting is impossible and concentration is facilitated. It promotes incredible flexibility of the hips, knees and ankles.

5　Lotus Position with Twist

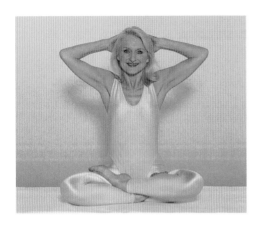

1 Sit in either a cross-legged, Half or Full Lotus Position. Interlock your hands behind your head.

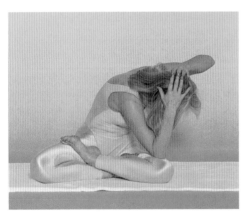

2 Take a deep breath in and as you exhale, gently take your right elbow to your left knee. Lifting your left elbow, aim to look behind you and, breathing normally, hold this position for a count of 5. Then gently return to an upright position.

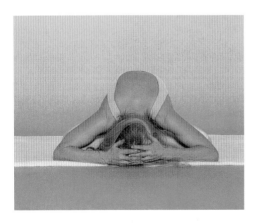

3 Repeat on the other side, then take a very deep breath and, as you exhale, gently bend forwards aiming your head to the floor. Breathing normally, relax in this position for a count of 5.

Inhale and return to an upright position, exhale and relax. Repeat the entire sequence twice.

Benefits
This is great for toning your midriff and waistline. It also removes tension from the lower back and increases spinal flexibility.

6   Back Stretch

This is a yoga essential. It is perfect for stretching and realigning the spine, and for toning the back and the thighs.

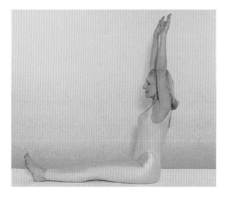

1 Sit very straight with both legs straight out in front of you. Take a deep breath in and lift both your arms straight up in the air.

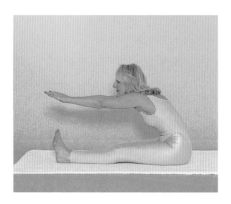

2 Exhale as you gradually bend forwards with your head up and back straight, eventually aiming your chin to your knees.

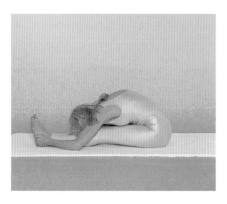

3 When you first start this movement, you will probably find that your chin and knees are a long way apart. Don't be discouraged – just keep practising.

Breathing normally, stay in your maximum position for a count of 5, then inhale, slowly lift your head and arms and return to an upright position. Exhale and relax. Repeat the movement twice.

Benefits
The Back Stretch releases tension in the lower back, stretches the hamstrings and tones the back of the thighs. It also tones the abdominal area, rejuvenates the entire spine and massages the heart. It is very relaxing.

7   Simple Twist

Please do not attempt if you are pregnant

This movement ensures flexibility of the spine and is excellent for slimming the midriff and waistline.

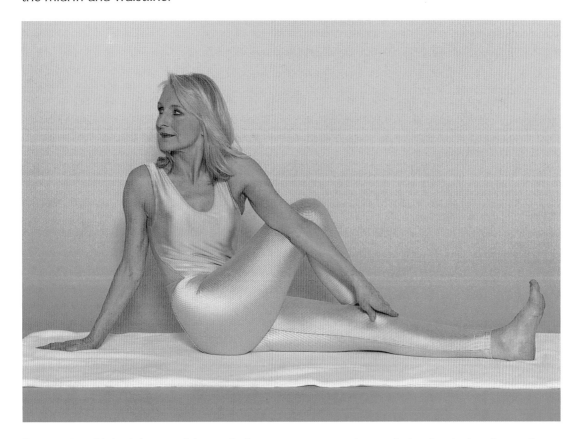

Sit straight with both legs straight out in front of you. Inhale deeply and, as you exhale, lift your right foot over your left leg, placing it on the floor on the outside of your left thigh. Place the right hand on the floor behind you.

Now, take your left arm and place it on the outside of your right knee and place your left hand on your left knee. Don't worry if you cannot quite reach, just let the hand rest where it is comfortable.

Take a deep breath in and, as you exhale, carefully twist your body to the right. Breathing normally, hold this position for a count of 5, increasing to 10 as you progress. Slowly return to the front. Repeat to the left and then repeat the entire movement once.

Benefits
This incredible movement releases tension from the spine and tones the spinal nerves. It is an excellent massage for the abdominal organs and stimulates circulation to the liver, spleen and kidneys. It is also a powerful toner for the midriff and waistline, hips and buttocks. It is also a great help when parking your car!

8   Wide-angled Leg Stretch

This is amazing for your shape! It tones the inner thighs, firms the midriff and waistline, and is great for ensuring flexibility in your lower back.

Sit straight with both your legs straight out in front of you. Spread them wide apart, making sure your hips feel comfortable when you do this. It is quite difficult to open them very wide at first, but flexibility will come with practise and perseverance. It is useful to gently massage your inner thighs before you start this movement to warm and relax your muscles.

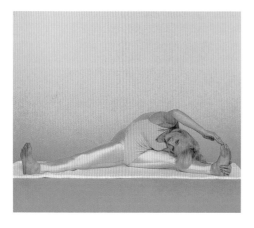

1 Take a deep breath and gently slide your right hand towards your right ankle, gradually lifting your left arm while aiming your left hand to your right foot and your right ear towards your right knee. Halfway is fine to start with.

Hold your maximum position for a count of 5, then inhale and slowly and gracefully return to an upright position. Repeat to the other side and then repeat the entire movement.

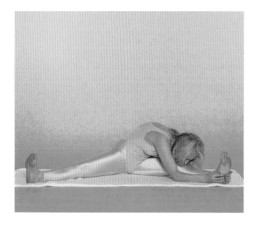

2 With both legs comfortably wide apart, breathe in and place both arms parallel to your right leg.

As you exhale, gently bend forwards, keeping your back flat, and aiming to clasp your right foot in both hands and then aim your chin towards your knee. Relax in your maximum position without strain, holding for a count of 5.

Taking a deep breath in, gently return to a sitting position, exhale, relax and repeat on the other side. Repeat the entire sequence twice.

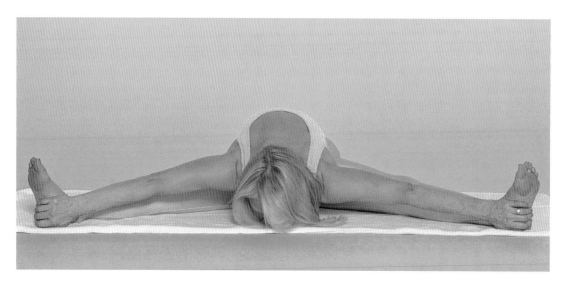

3 With both legs comfortably wide apart, place your arms parallel to your legs.

Inhale deeply and, as you exhale, keeping your head up and your back straight, move calmly and carefully into your maximum forwards stretch without strain. Don't worry if you do not get far in the beginning. Patience, perseverance and daily practice

always work and your chin will eventually be on the floor! Remain in your maximum position for a count of 5, increasing to a count of 10 as you progress.

Inhale and, lifting your head and arms gently, return to an upright position. Exhale and relax. Repeat the movement 3 times.

Benefits
As well as being a powerful toner for your thighs, midriff and waistline, this movement is extremely good for relieving tension in the lower back. It can be most beneficial for people suffering from sciatica. It relieves tension in the lower abdominal area and can assist tremendously with menstrual problems.

9 Full Twist

Please do not attempt if you are pregnant

Do not attempt this movement until you can do the Simple Twist with ease.

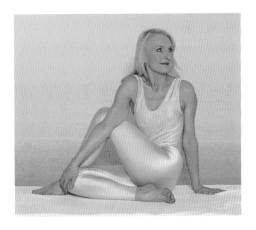

1 Sit with both legs straight out in front of you and bring your right heel next to your groin.

Place your left hand on the floor behind your back. Bring your left foot over your right thigh and place it on the floor alongside the thigh.

Now take a deep breath and, as you exhale, take your right arm on the outside of the left knee and place it on your right knee, gently twisting the body, turning the head over the left shoulder. Breathing normally, hold this position for a count of 5, increasing to a count of 10 as you progress.

Advanced Full Twist

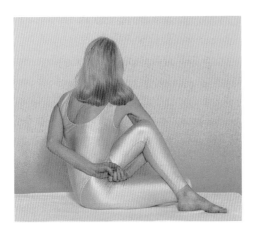

2 For a more advanced stretch in your maximum twist, slide your right hand under your left knee and take your left hand behind your back and try to join your hands together, holding for a count of 5.

Release and inhale, then return your head to the front. Unclasp your hands and relax. Repeat on the other side and then repeat the entire sequence just once.

Benefits
The Full Twist has all the benefits of the simple twist. It creates amazing flexibility in the spine, shoulders, elbows, wrists, fingers, hips, knees, ankles and toes. It is also great for firming the neck, jaw and throat. It is complicated, but I promise you that it is worth it!

10 Pose of a Cobra

This is one of the best movements for keeping the spine in perfect condition. It greatly increases spinal strength and flexibility.

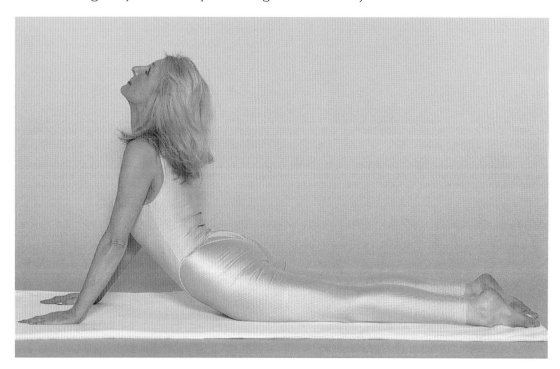

Lie face downwards on the mat with your forehead on the floor and your hands 3 inches from your body, in line with your shoulders, fingertips pointing forwards.

Inhale deeply and, as you exhale, gently lift your head and place your chin on the floor. Inhale again and, keeping your lower abdomen on the floor, lift your upper body. Come up into your maximum position. Eventually you will be able to straighten your arms and stretch your body backwards. Don't be disappointed if this doesn't happen at first. Halfway is fine for the moment. Breathing normally, hold your maximum position for a count of 5, increasing to 10 as you progress.

Slowly lower yourself to the floor, place your head on the floor then turn your head to one side and relax. Repeat this movement just once. Lift your bottom in the air and slowly take it down to your heels, stretching your arms forwards into the Pose of a Swan.

Benefits
This is excellent for toning and firming the muscles of the throat and jaw. It tones the upper arms, corrects poor posture, tones the bust and is excellent for relieving menstrual problems such as cramps and backache. It tones the liver and spleen and is beneficial for people with backache and arthritis. It also stretches out the spine and gives it tremendous flexibility.

11 Pose of a Cat

Every animal on this planet stretches after a rest to ensure its spine is free from tension and ready for action. We can really help ourselves if we stretch as well.

Stage one

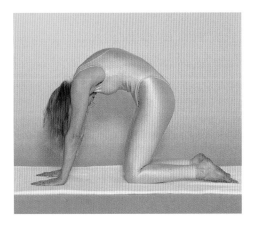

1 Adopt an all fours position with your knees, feet and hands all about a foot apart. Ensure that your thighs are vertical with your hips, straight above your knees, and your shoulders are straight above your wrists.

Arch your back into a hump, at the same time dropping your head.

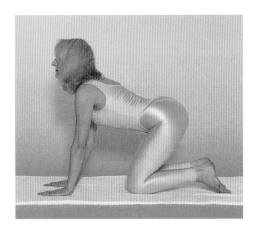

2 Slowly lift your head and lower the small of your back so that your bottom sticks out. Drop your head and arch your back and continue moving your back this way until you have done it at least 5 times. This part of the movement is a great way to rid the spine of tension.

Stage two

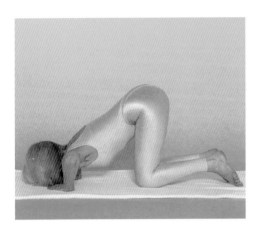

1 After releasing the tension in your spine in Stage one, and still on all fours, bend your elbows and place your chin on the floor. Hold this position for a count of 2.

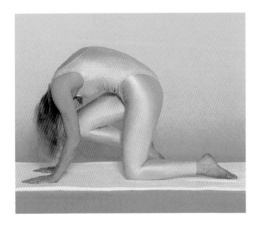

2 Straighten your arms and gently lift your right knee, aiming it to touch your forehead.

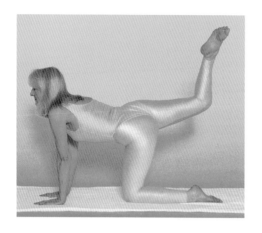

3 Slowly lift your head and swing your right leg up behind you, aiming to point your toes to the ceiling while looking at the ceiling at the same time. Repeat this sequence 3 times and then do it 3 times on the other side.

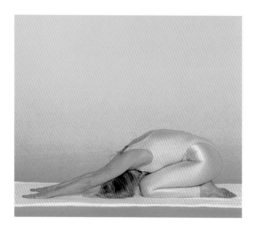

4 Finish by inhaling deeply, then lowering your bottom to your heels as you exhale, keeping your arms straight out in front of you. Relax in this beautiful stretch called the Pose of a Swan for a count of 5.

Inhale, return to a kneeling position and stretch your arms up straight above your head. Hold this stretch for a count of 5, then exhale and relax.

Benefits
This gives a powerful tension release to the entire spine and it is really helpful for aching backs. It tones and firms the wrists, arms, thighs and bottom.

12 Pose of a Camel

This movement is another wonderful backward stretch. It releases all tensions, so your cares just slip away!

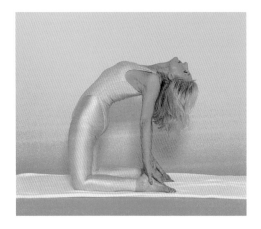

1 Adopt a high kneeling position with your knees and feet 1 foot apart. Place your hands at your waistline with your thumbs in front and fingers behind. Take a deep breath in and with full lungs, gently relax backwards keeping your thighs straight. Arch backwards to your maximum position, aiming the palms of your hands flat on your feet.

If you cannot yet reach, keep your hands at your waistline and stay in your maximum position, breathing normally for a count of 5. If you can place your hands on your feet, well done!

From this position, take a deep breath and exhale fully, push your abdomen, thighs and hips forwards, at the same time arching your torso as far back as possible for a fantastic stretch. Hold this position for a count of 5, increasing to 10 as you progress.

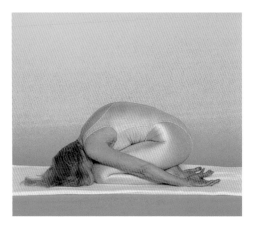

2 Inhale as you slowly come into an upright position, then exhale and lower your bottom to your heels, placing your hands by your sides, and relax in the Pose of a Child.

Inhale, return to the high kneeling position, and repeat the movement once.

Benefits
This movement tones the thighs, midriff and waistline. It greatly expands the chest and is very helpful to people with asthma and other breathing problems. It also firms the jaw and the throat, corrects poor posture and relaxes your whole body.

13 Pose of a Dog

We can learn so much from watching animals! This incredible stretch is excellent for removing tension from your spine and it can help people with lower backache and shoulder tension. Do not attempt the Pose of a Dog until you feel quite comfortable with the Pose of a Cobra.

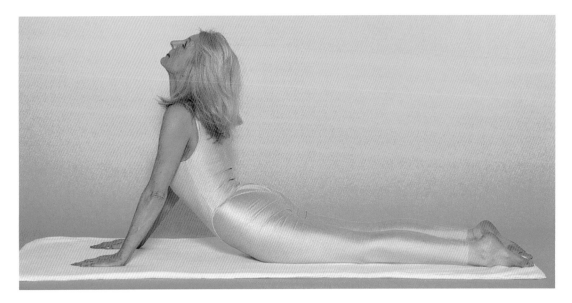

Lie face down on the mat with your hands on either side at shoulder level, fingertips facing forwards. Inhale deeply and, keeping your lower abdomen on the floor, slowly come up into the Pose of a Cobra. Breathing normally, hold for a count of 5.

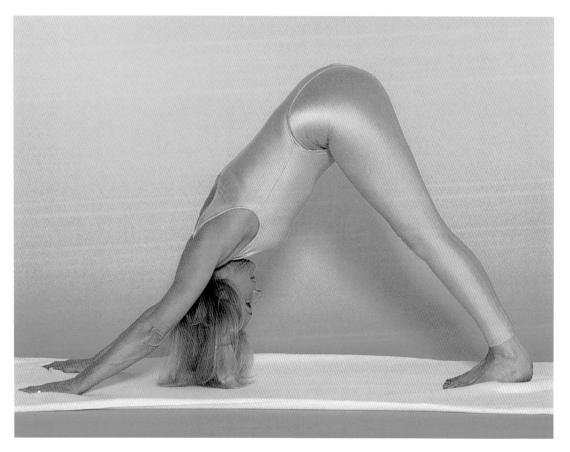

Exhale and, tucking your toes under, push down on your hands, lift your bottom in the air and push your heels down towards the floor, taking your head down between your arms so that your body resembles an inverted 'V'. Again, this is not easy at first – just do your best. Breathing normally, hold this position for a count of 5, then slowly swing your head back between your arms and gently lower your body to the floor and relax.

Repeat this powerful stretch just once to begin, building up to performing the entire movement 3 times as your strength increases.

Benefits

As well as having all the benefits of the Pose of a Cobra, this position increases the flexibility of the spine, hamstrings and calf muscles. It strengthens the arms and relieves tension in the lower back, neck and shoulders.

14 Pose of a Rabbit

An excellent movement for relieving tension from the neck and stimulating blood flow to the brain.

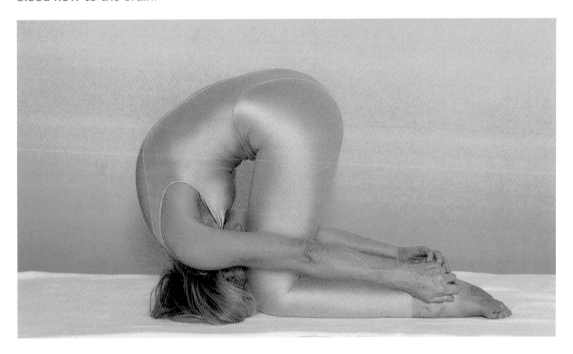

Kneel with your bottom on your heels and place your forehead on the floor. Place your hands on your heels.

Inhale and, as you exhale, place your forehead on your knees. Gripping your heels firmly with your hands, gently lift your bottom in the air, aiming to have your arms straight and your thighs perpendicular to the floor.

To accomplish this you may have to nudge your knees gently towards your forehead. This can take a while, so don't strain – just take it carefully.

Make sure your body weight is supported by your arms stretching back to your heels with only a fraction of the weight on your head.

Hold your maximum position for a count of 5, increasing to 10 as you progress. Inhale and slowly lower your bottom to your heels and relax in the Pose of a Child. Hold for a count of 10, then slowly return to a sitting position and relax, lying down for a count of 10. Do not repeat.

Benefits
This is a wonderful tension release for the neck and spine and is a great help to headache sufferers. It is very beneficial for the skin and hair due to the increased circulation of blood in those areas. It stimulates the thyroid and parathyroid glands in the neck and is most beneficial to the sinuses.

I5   Alternate Nostril Breathing Exercise

This is so soothing and it will help you stay calm and peaceful during stressful times. It is ideal to do at night before you go to sleep, but equally it will help you cope with any tense or upsetting situations.

One of my pupils, an English teacher in a girls' school, has had incredible results with using this breathing exercise to calm her pupils down before their exams.

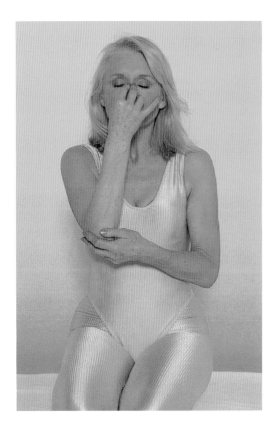

Sit straight in a kneeling or cross-legged position. Place your right thumb on your right nostril. Place your next two fingers on the bridge of your nose and your next finger on your left nostril. Place your left hand under your right elbow to support it.

Unblock your right nostril by lifting your thumb and inhale through it for a count of 5. Block your right nostril with your thumb and hold your breath for a count of 5 then slowly unblock the left nostril and exhale calmly and slowly for a count of 5.

Inhale through the left nostril for a count of 5, hold your breath for a count of 5 and then exhale through your right nostril for a count of 5. Continue this cycle for 10 rounds.

Benefits
This is a wonderful tranquillizer and is excellent for helping you cope with life's pressures. It is also of great help to those who suffer from congested sinuses.

16 Head and Neck Exercises

Please do not attempt if you have neck problems

A great tension release for the proverbial 'pain in the neck'. I have not seen as many tense and tight necks in my 30 years of teaching yoga as I have in the last 3 years!

Go gently with this movement, making the tiniest movements to start with and then gradually increasing the movement as your neck becomes easier. Never strain!

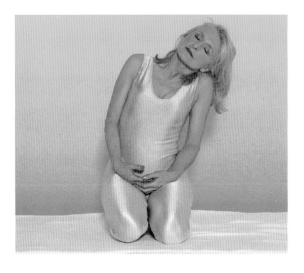

1 Sit with your back straight in either a cross-legged or kneeling position. Gently drop your head forwards then slowly roll it to the right.

2 Gently allow your head to roll back. Roll your head slowly to the left and then slowly and carefully forwards. Make 3 slow gentle circles to the right and then gently rotate the head the other way round, making 3 circles to the left.

Benefits
This movement, as well as releasing tension from the neck, helps remove the calcium deposits that can settle on the joint surfaces, so alleviating tightness and stiffness in the neck. It is excellent in helping to remove a double chin, toning and firming the muscles of the jaw and throat. If you are having a hard day, it is a good idea to stop and do the movement in your office to relieve the tension build up in your neck. It is really beneficial for headache and migraine sufferers.

17 The Plough

Please do not attempt if you are pregnant

Please do not attempt if you have high blood pressure

This beautifully relaxing position stretches out the spine, stimulates blood flow to the head and neck area, so nourishing your skin, hair and brain cells.

Stage one

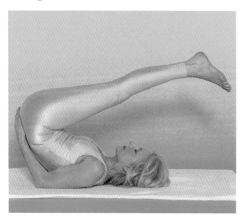

1 Lie down with your back on the mat. Inhale and bend your knees, gently lifting your bottom from the floor as far as you can, but making sure that you don't strain. Place your hands on your lower back to give support and aim to have your legs parallel to the floor.

This is Stage one of the Plough. Hold this movement for just 10 seconds to begin with, building up very gradually until you are able to stay there for 30 seconds.

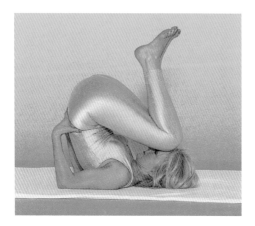

2 Gently draw your knees to your forehead then very slowly roll down your spine, just a vertebra at a time, until your bottom touches the floor.

Interlock your hands around your knees, then gently rock from side to side, relaxing your back into the floor. Lie down on your back, breathe slowly and deeply, and relax.

Stage two

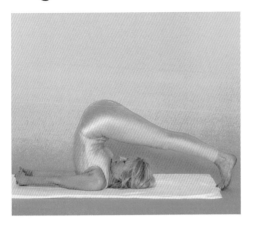

3 As you progress you will find that the movement eases tension in your lower back and gradually your feet will be able to touch the floor. When this happens you no longer need your hands to support your back, so stretch them in the opposite direction to your feet. Interlock them and enjoy the lovely stretch.

Breathing normally, hold the position for 30 seconds and, supporting your back, roll down in exactly the same way as in Stage one.

A longer stay in it is a wonderful stress reliever. I recommend increasing the hold by 30 seconds per week until you are able to hold it for up to 3 minutes.

All men's miseries derive from not being able to sit quiet in a room alone.
BLAISE PASCAL, *Pensées*

Benefits
An amazing movement – it releases tension in the lower back and can help to relieve backache. It stimulates blood flow to the thyroid and parathyroid glands in the neck, helping to keep them in excellent condition. By stimulating blood flow to the head and neck area, it boosts the condition of the skin and hair and so is very rejuvenating.

18 Pose of a Fish

This pose relaxes the chest and neck and is great to do after both the Plough and the Shoulderstand.

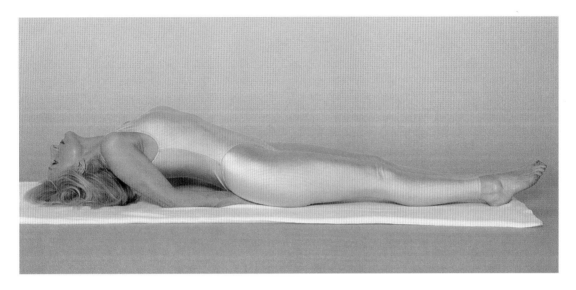

Lie flat on your back. Place your hands facing downwards under your buttocks with your elbows bent so that the lower arms support the upper body.

Inhale gently and lift your head, arching backwards so that the chest is arched and the top of the head is on the floor. Breathe slowly and deeply in this position and hold it for a count of 3 deep breaths to begin with, gradually increasing to 5 as you progress.

Gently remove your hands, then slowly lie down flat on your back and relax.

Benefits
A lovely relaxing movement, this tones and firms the throat and jaw, and tones the thyroid and parathyroid glands in the neck. It is excellent for relieving tension in the neck, carefully expands the chest and is beneficial to people who suffer from chesty conditions and asthma.

19 Deep Relaxation

At the end of your exercises, take time out to relax both your body and mind. Lie flat on the mat and ensure that you are warm enough (your body temperature can drop when you relax). It is a good idea to cover yourself with a blanket in cold weather.

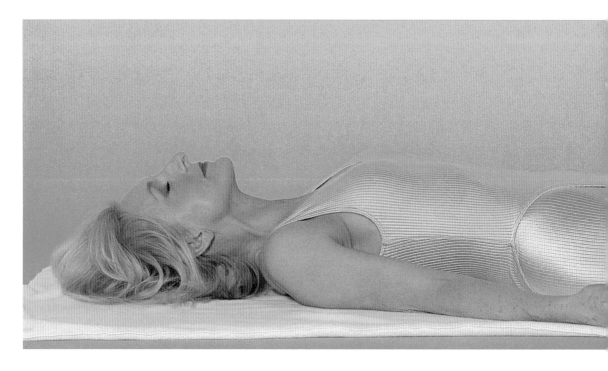

Have your legs about 2 feet apart and your arms about 1 foot from your body with your palms facing upwards. Slow your breathing down, inhaling and exhaling slowly and peacefully through your nose.

Now relax each part of your body in turn.

o Relax your feet, ankles and calves.
o Relax your thighs and feel your legs becoming heavy, limp and totally relaxed.
o Relax your lower abdominal muscles, then your back and your chest.
o Feel your shoulders relaxing, and your arms and your hands.

Now feel your entire arms becoming heavy and limp.

- Relax your neck and your facial muscles, letting your jaw become limp and heavy.
- Let your eyelids feel heavy and your eyeballs roll upwards.
- Let your scalp slide back and feel your entire body relaxing deeply into the floor.

Allow yourself to feel dreamy and drowsy, making sure that all negative thoughts leave your mind. Fill your mind with a wonderful feeling of gratitude for all your many blessings.

Now relax into a lovely feeling of peace, calm and happiness. While your body is relaxed, visualize a beautiful clear night sky. See a full moon shining on still water. Now watch the silvery moonlight. Relax, relax, relax! Stay relaxed for 5–15 minutes, then take a deep breath, stretch your arms back behind your head, and breathe in energy and that good-to-be-alive feeling. Exhale and relax. Inhale and slowly come up into a sitting position.

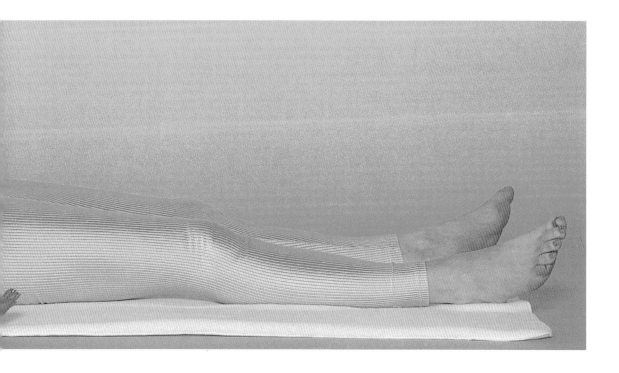

Benefits
Chronic tension literally strangles the body, inhibiting the flow of blood and lymph to the tissues. In time, this can weaken the body and lead to disease. When the tension has been removed from your body, it is much easier to relax both body and mind. This results in an increased blood flow to all tissues, so allowing them all the nutrients they require. As the lymphatic system becomes free of tension, waste products are gently removed from your system. When the mind is clear, peaceful and calm, your problems seem easier to solve. New ideas arrive and the way ahead becomes clearer. You will discover the inner calm and happiness that has always been within you.

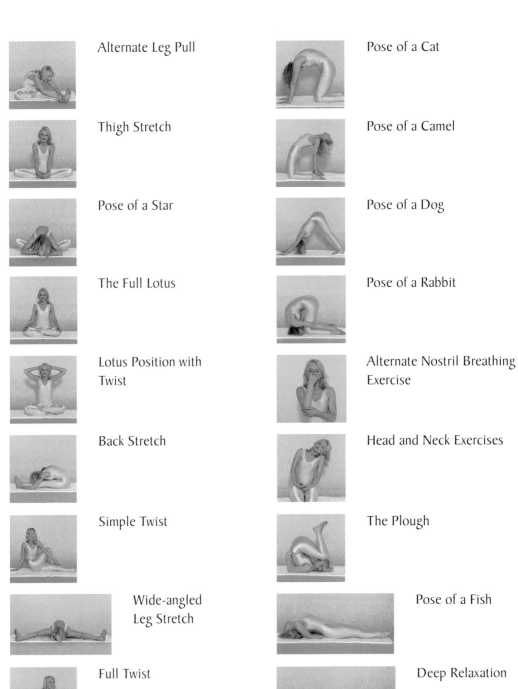

Alternate Leg Pull

Pose of a Cat

Thigh Stretch

Pose of a Camel

Pose of a Star

Pose of a Dog

The Full Lotus

Pose of a Rabbit

Lotus Position with Twist

Alternate Nostril Breathing Exercise

Back Stretch

Head and Neck Exercises

Simple Twist

The Plough

Wide-angled Leg Stretch

Pose of a Fish

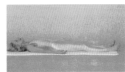

Full Twist

Deep Relaxation

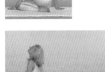

Pose of a Cobra

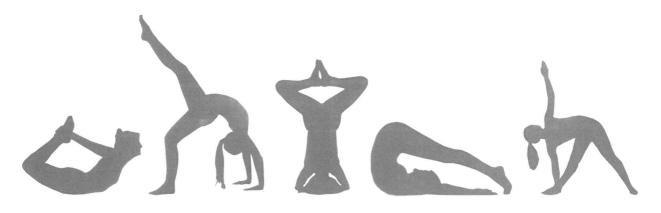

advanced class

> **CAUTION:**
>
> Please do not attempt any of the movements
> in this chapter during pregnancy.

It is incredibly exciting to progress in yoga and to rediscover your energy and flexibility. It is wonderful to be able to improve at something physical as you grow older and all this can bring new confidence. Here, I offer you a slightly stronger sequence of movements so that you can develop even further.

Please don't be tempted to start this chapter until you are comfortable with the preceding movements. As ever, always move carefully and do not strain. Because I have aimed to give you an enjoyable, yet balanced session, I have included some relatively easy movements along with the more advanced ones. Above all, enjoy this session!

chapter eight

I   Salute to the Sun

Please do not attempt if you are pregnant

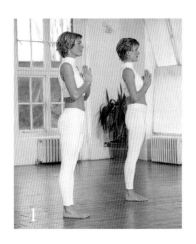
1

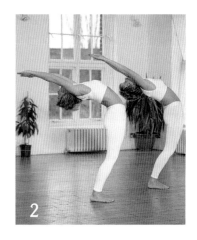
2

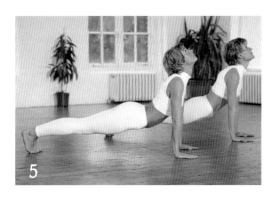
5

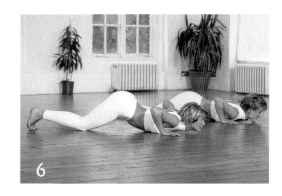
6

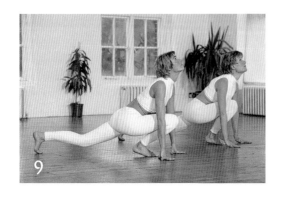
9

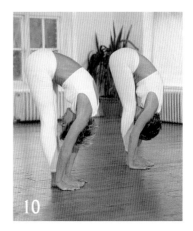
10

From now on, start every new day with this energizing sequence. We practised this in the Advanced Ten-minute Miracle (see page 16), but as you perform the movements now, aim to move with much more flexibility in each posture. When Salute to the Sun becomes much easier for you, then perform it with your feet together for a stronger stretch.

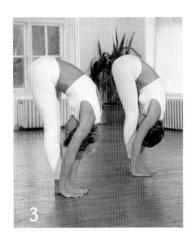

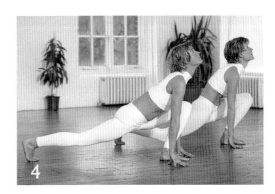

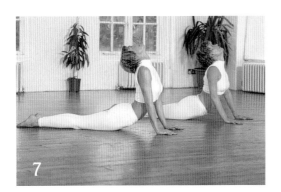

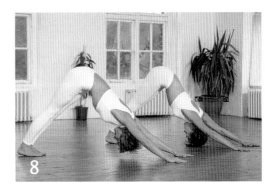

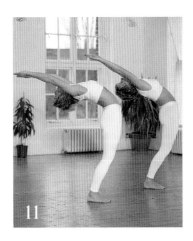

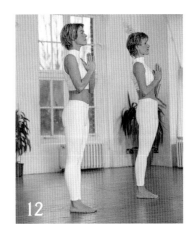

2 Straight Leg Triangle

Please do not attempt if you are pregnant

A total body toner.

Stage one

1 Stand straight in perfect posture with your feet together. Inhale and place your legs 3–4 feet apart. As you exhale, turn your right foot at an angle of 90° to the right and move your arms parallel to the floor.

Inhale deeply and, as you exhale, keep the knees straight and aim your right hand flat on the floor by your right foot, with your little finger by your big toe. If you cannot do this yet, then hold your right leg wherever it is comfortable, but do

not bend the right knee.
Gently stretch your left arm up in the air, pulling your shoulder back to open the chest, and look at your left hand. Hold the pose for a count of 5, increasing to 10 as you progress.

Breathe normally in your maximum position. Inhale slowly and return to an upright position. Exhale, relax and repeat this movement with the left foot at a 90° angle to the left side. Repeat the entire movement once.

Stage two

1 Stand with your legs about 3–4 feet apart, ensuring that your knees are straight. Inhale and rotate your right foot 90° to the right, keeping your left foot facing forwards. Place your arms parallel to the floor.

2 Inhale deeply and, as you exhale, change your arms over so that the left hand is pointing towards the right foot.

3 Inhale and, as you exhale, keep your knees straight and bend forwards, aiming your left thumb by your right big toe and the palm of the hand flat on the floor. In the beginning stages, ensure both knees are straight and place the left hand on the right leg wherever it is comfortable.

4 Slowly draw your right arm up in the air, aiming to have it in a straight line with your left arm, then carefully rotate your trunk so that you are looking at your right hand. Breathing normally, hold this position for a count of 5, increasing the hold to a count of 10 as you progress.

5 Inhale and lift the left hand up from the floor. Carefully return your upper body to an upright position. Exhale and repeat the pose on the left side, turning the left foot at a 90° angle to the left. Repeat the entire sequence once.

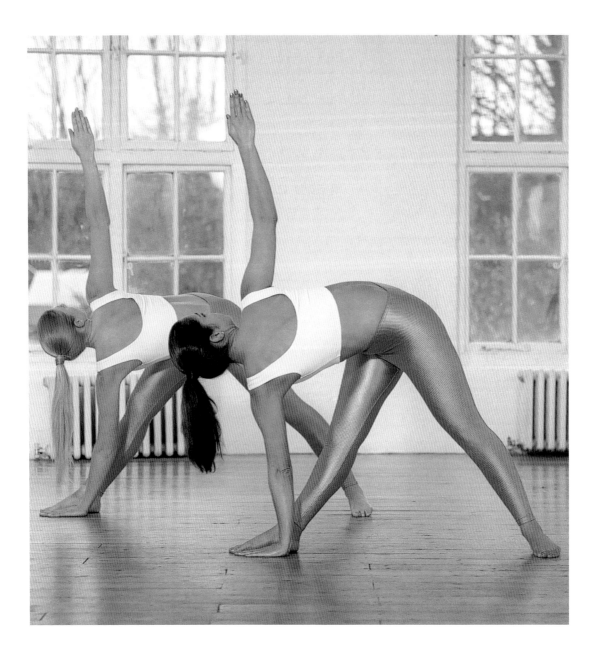

Stage three

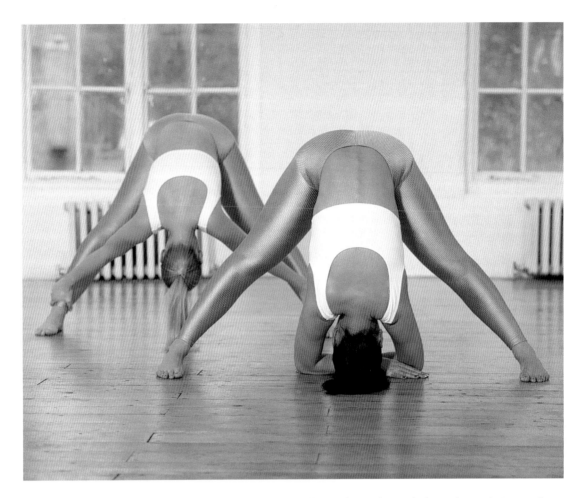

1 With your legs 3 feet apart and both feet facing forwards, take a deep breath in, stretch your arms up in the air and, as you exhale, stretch forwards with your back flat and legs straight. Relax in your maximum forwards stretch, clasping your legs with your hands. Breathing normally, hold this position for a count of 5.

At the end of this hold, try this extra stretch, but only when you feel you are ready for it.

Spread your legs a little wider and aim to place your head on the floor. Do not strain. Eventually you will be able to relax, fold your arms and rest your head on your folded arms. Hold again for a count of 5 in your maximum position, then inhale and slowly bring your feet inwards until they are about 3 feet apart. Return to an upright position, lifting your head first and keeping your back straight, then stretch your arms above your head, exhale and relax.

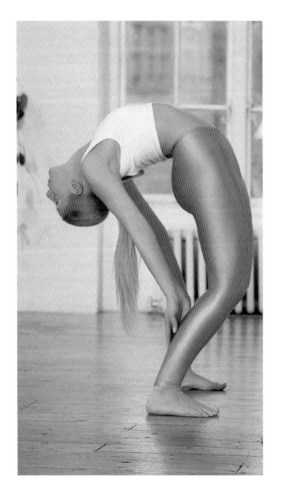

2 Now place your hands on your waistline with your thumbs in front and your fingers at the back, keeping your legs about 3 feet apart. Inhale deeply and slowly and then, as you exhale, bend backwards in your maximum position. Hold for a count of 5 and, if you feel comfortable in the backwards stretch, move your hands down and aim to touch your calves. Don't strain, the flexibility will come with the '3 Ps' – patience, practice and perseverance. Inhale, slowly return to an upright position and exhale. There is no need to repeat this sequence.

Benefits

I don't think you need me to tell you that the Straight Leg Triangle sequence firms and tones virtually every muscle in your body.

Stage one is especially good for toning the leg muscles and relieving tension in the lower back and the chest. It dramatically increases your flexibility and is an excellent help for people with lower backache.

Stage two is excellent for toning and firming the buttocks and calves, and for stretching the hamstrings. Again, it is excellent for the lumbar spine and is a boon to people with lower backache. It tones the abdominal organs and increases shoulder flexibility.

Stage three stimulates blood flow to the head and neck area, thus helping the skin, hair and brain cells. It is excellent for stretching and toning the hamstrings and adductor muscles. The backwards stretch relieves tightness in the chest and is beneficial to the lungs. It corrects poor posture and is excellent for the flexibility of the spine. It also tones the neck, jaw and throat.

3   Standing Head to Knee Posture

An excellent balance to tone the thighs and keep the back flexible.

Stand straight with your feet together. Inhale and lift your right leg with your knee bent, interlocking your hands under your right foot.

Stare at a spot on the floor and carefully start to stretch your right leg, aiming to have it straight, and then gently draw your chin to your knee. Your left leg should remain completely straight throughout. Breathing normally, hold for your maximum position for a count of 5, increasing to 10 as you progress.

Gently release your hold on your leg, lower it, then stand up straight and relax. Repeat with the other leg and then repeat the entire movement once.

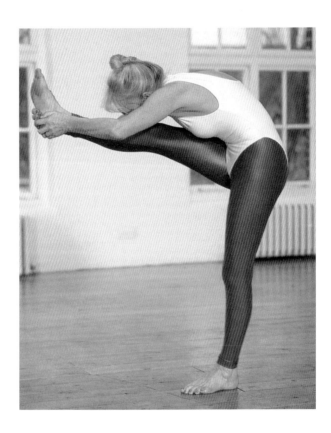

Benefits
This really takes your mind off everything because you have to concentrate enormously on the job in hand. Physically, it tones your thighs, stretches your hamstrings and releases tension in your lower back. It is an excellent strengthener for the leg you are standing on. Do it daily and watch the cellulite disappear.

4　Pose of a Tree

Yoga teaches us to look to the willow tree for an example on how to cope with the storms in life. The willow, being flexible, bends in the storm and although it may lose some twigs and leaves, it generally copes and survives. The oak, on the other hand, although much stronger and sturdier that the willow, is extremely rigid and often falls in a storm. Yoga teaches us to be like the willow and keep our bodies and minds flexible, able to cope with the mental and physical storms that life throws at us. The Pose of a Tree is excellent for our poise, balance, concentration and flexibility.

Stage one

We first practised this in detail in Chapter 3 (see page 30). It was probably quite difficult when you started this movement, but I am sure it is much easier now.

1　Inhale, keeping your eyes on a spot to aid your balance, gently lift your right foot on to your left thigh with the sole of the foot facing the ceiling. Don't worry if you cannot do this yet. Just place your foot on your ankle, calf or knee and progress at your own pace.

2　Having selected a position for your foot, inhale deeply and stretch both your arms above your head, placing the palms of your hands together.

3　Staring at your spot and breathing normally, hold for a count of 5, lengthening the count to 10 as you progress. Now, if you are staying with Stage one for the moment, take your foot down and repeat the movement on the other side. Then repeat the entire sequence.

Please do not attempt if you are pregnant

Stage two

Do not move on to Stage two until you can perform Stage one correctly and easily.

1　With your foot comfortably on your upper thigh, stare at a spot on the floor. Inhale deeply and, keeping your eyes on your spot, start to bend forwards aiming your hands to the floor and, eventually, your chin to your knee. Just do your best, halfway down is fine at first.

2　Now, keeping your eyes on your spot, lift your head and then gradually lift the upper body. Concentrate hard on your spot and then carefully return to an upright position.

3　Stretch your arms up in the air and then exhale. Gently take your foot down and relax. Repeat to the other side just once.

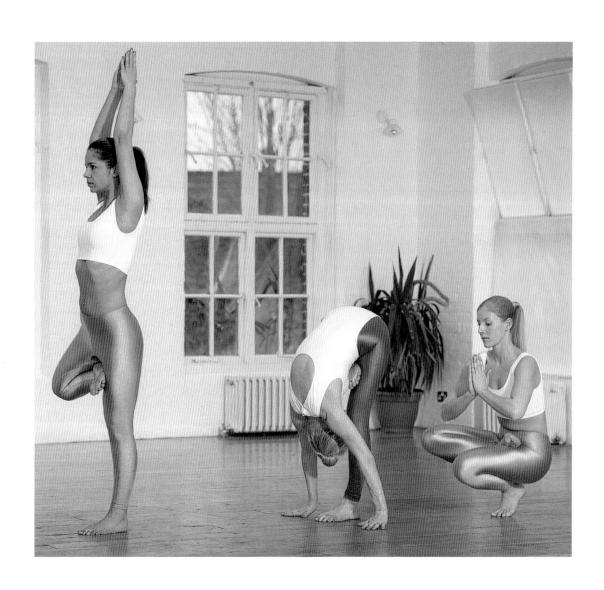

Stage three

Please wait until you can perform both Stages one and two with ease before attempting Stage three. Then, as always, proceed with caution.

1 Stand straight and place your right foot on your left thigh as in Stage one. Inhale deeply, lifting your arms above your head and, as you slowly exhale with flat back and straight leg, move forward into Stage two.

2 Ensuring that you concentrate on your spot, place your hands on the floor and aim your head to your knee. Find another spot and transfer your weight onto your hands, and aim to bend your left knee and gently lower your left buttock to your left heel while keeping your hands on the floor. Be extremely careful and ensure that you keep your weight on your hands.

3 When your left buttock is comfortably on your left heel, and only if you feel ready, lift your hands from the floor and place them either in prayer or on your left knee. Keep your eyes on your spot. Hold for a count of 1 at first, increasing to 5 as you progress.

4 To come out of this position, place your hands on the floor in front of you and push forward so that once again your weight is on your hands.

Bend forward so that you are able to straighten your left leg, then slowly lift your head. Inhaling deeply, come back up into an upright position. Stretch your arms above your head, exhale, relax and repeat to the other side. Relax and do not repeat the movement. Massage your knees gently – you and they deserve it.

Benefits
When starting yoga, even the Pose of a Tree – Stage one can be very difficult. Pupils often say that their leggings are too slippery and the foot will not stay up, but this is not the case – the problem is stiffness in the hip, knee or ankle. At 29, my knees were incredibly stiff and I know the problem all too well. I hated this movement and over the years I have watched many pupils discover that their joints are also remarkably stiff. But yoga does work quickly and I promise you that if you obey the rules, progress calmly and always without strain, you will be amazed at the way your joints rediscover their natural flexibility. The movement also tones the inner and outer thighs, corrects posture and aids concentration.

Stages two and three will keep your legs in incredible condition, helping the flexibility of all your joints. They are excellent for your concentration, patience and perseverance as they totally take your mind off your daily life. They firm and tone all the muscles in your legs, giving them a beautiful toned shape whatever your age. Believe me it is worth it!

5 Pose of a Sage

A strong twist to remove tension from the spine and to slim and firm the midriff and waistline.

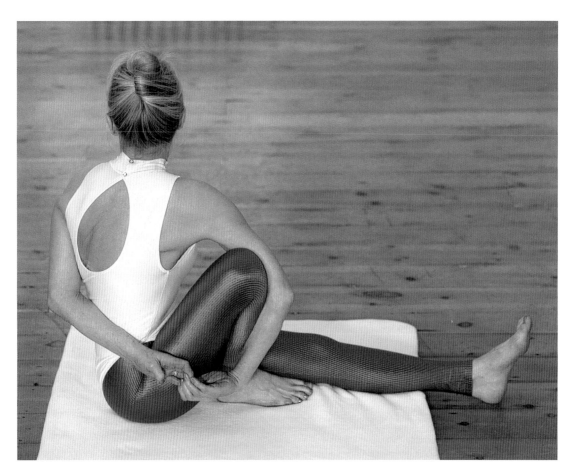

1 Sit straight with both legs straight out in front of you. Place your right foot by your right buttock. Inhaling deeply, place your right arm on the inside of your right knee. Exhaling, take your left arm behind your back and, sitting completely straight aim to join your hands together. Don't worry if you can't do this at first. Stay sitting straight keeping your hands in their maximum position. Inhale deeply and, as you exhale, slowly turn your head over your left shoulder, again ensuring that your spine is straight. Breathing normally, hold this position for a count of 5, then slowly return your head to the front, facing forwards over your left leg.

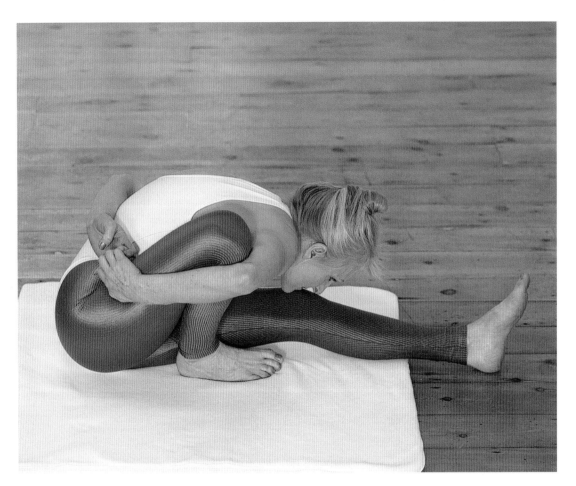

2 Inhale and, keeping your arms entwined around your right knee, exhale and slowly stretch forwards keeping your head up, your back flat and your leg straight. With your back flat, gently draw your chin to your left knee or your maximum position without strain. Breathing normally, hold for a count of 5. Inhale and return to an upright position. Exhale, relax and repeat to the other side. Repeat the entire movement just once.

Benefits

This is excellent for the lower back and it greatly helps people with lower backache. As we discover so often in yoga movements, one side of our body is much more flexible than the other. We can help the spine enormously by carefully sorting out these imbalances. This movement can help relieve shoulder tension, and firm and tone the midriff, waistline, jaw and throat. Internally, it will tone the liver and spleen.

6　Back Stretch

Please do not attempt if you are pregnant

After finishing the Pose of a Sage, which works each side of the body separately, it is always a good idea to follow with the Back Stretch to help rebalance the spine. We first learnt this movement in Chapter 7 (see page 82). Here it is again.

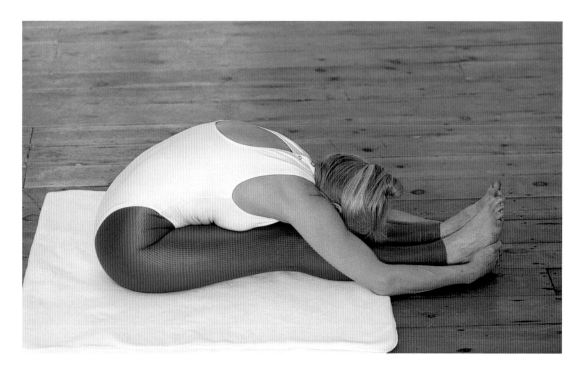

Sit straight with your legs together, straight out in front of you.

Inhale deeply and lift your arms above your head. Exhale as you slowly and carefully stretch forwards with your back straight and head up. Aim to clasp your feet and aim your chin to your knees, gently allowing your elbows to drop towards the floor while clasping your heels. Breathing normally, stay in your maximum position for a count of 10, exhale and try to relax down a little further without straining.

Inhale as you lift your head and gradually come up into a sitting position. Stretch your arms up above your head and relax. Repeat 3 times.

Benefits
The Back Stretch releases tension in the lower back, stretches the hamstrings and tones the back of the thighs. It also tones the abdominal area, rejuvenates the entire spine and massages the heart. It is very relaxing.

7   Pose of a Bow

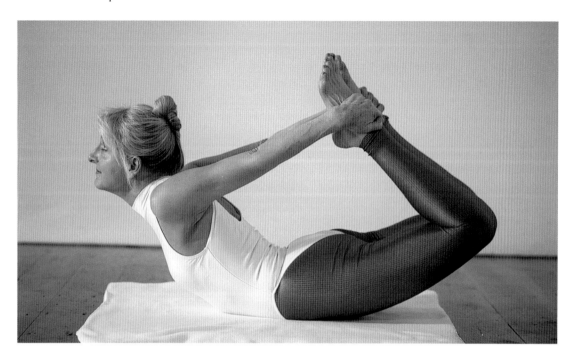

Please do not attempt if you are pregnant

A beautiful backwards bend to give great flexibility to the spine and help relieve digestive and menstrual problems.

Lie face down on your mat. Inhale and clasp the outside of your feet in your hands. If you cannot do this at first then put your socks on, let the toe loosen and grab the toes. Exhale and relax.

Take another breath and lift both your head and feet from the floor, stretching them upwards as high as you can go without strain. Exhale and stay in the maximum position, breathing normally, for a count of 5, increasing to 10 as you progress. Gently allow your body to return slowly to the floor. Unclasp your feet, turn your head on one side and relax. Repeat this movement once.

When, and only when, you feel confident in the Pose of a Bow, you can then try rocking forwards and backwards in your maximum position. Do this just three times to begin with and then gently release your feet, slowly lowering your body to the floor. Lie flat and relax. Do not repeat the rocking movement.

Benefits
This wonderful movement is very relaxing and is an ideal position to stretch away the cares of the day before going to sleep. It keeps your spine young and flexible and helps correct your posture. It tones the arms, throat, jaw and thighs and is a great help for women who suffer from menstrual cramps. It also improves digestion and strengthens the abdominal muscles.

8 Pose of a Tortoise

The ancient texts tell us that the sacred nectar with which the Gods preserved their youth had been lost. To retrieve this, one of the Gods, Visnu, turned himself into a huge tortoise and dived deep into the ocean to retrieve this precious nectar. The movement is dedicated to this tortoise. This is a most important movement in yoga. Once you have mastered it, you do feel as though you have had a spoonful of nectar! It is a most stimulating and refreshing movement and excellent for relieving lower back tension.

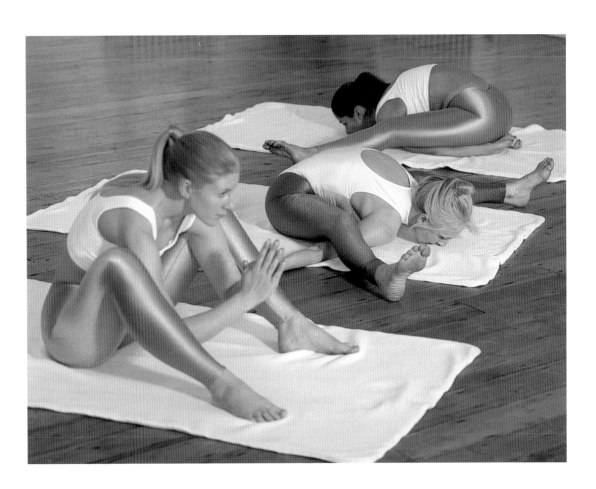

1 Sit on the floor with your legs bent and your feet about 1 foot apart with your feet facing outwards. Place your hands together in prayer. Inhale deeply and, as you exhale, gently draw your elbows to the floor.

2 Now open your arms and endeavour to stretch them under your legs and out the other side. In your maximum stretch, notice the position of your elbows. If they are on the outer side of your knee then you are ready to progress. If not, simply stay in this position and hold for a count of 5, then slowly inhale and return to an upright position. As you practise you will quickly improve, so don't worry.

3 If you have your elbows on the outer side of your knee, take a large breath, then, as you exhale, stretch your legs forward and outwards slowly and gently, aiming

to have your legs straight. At the same time, stretch your arms straight out at your sides and aim your chin to the floor. Be careful not to strain. Breathing normally, stay in this position for a count of 5, increasing to 10 as you progress.

4 Inhale and slowly bring your legs in first and then your arms as you return to an upright position. Once you have mastered the maximum position with ease, you may then like to try the next stage.

In your maximum position, slowly draw your arms behind your back and aim to clasp them together. Breathing normally, hold this position for a count of 10. Inhale, unclasp your arms, draw your feet towards your body and gently return to a sitting position. Exhale and relax.

Benefits
This posture gives you a lovely feeling of peace and calm. It soothes your nerves, tones and releases tension from your lower back, tones your abdominal organs and helps create flexibility in your hips.

9   Maltese Cross

This three-part sequence is wonderful for the shape of your thighs and bottom and is great for relieving stiffness and tension in the lower back and hips.

Stage one

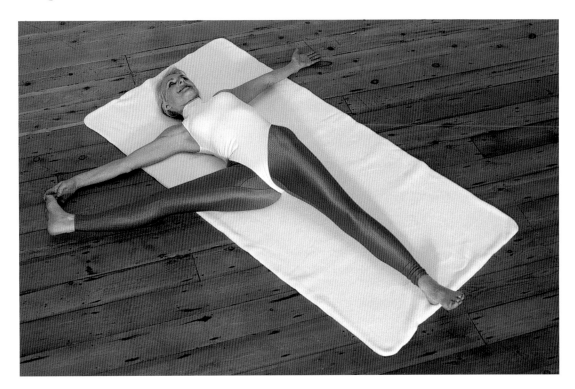

1   Lie flat on your back with your arms stretched out at shoulder level and your legs together so that you resemble a cross.

2   Inhale and, as you exhale, slowly stretch your right leg and, keeping your heel on the floor, aim your foot to your right hand. Your aim is to clasp your big toe! This sounds very easy but the heel must not leave the floor.

Don't worry if only a little movement is possible at first. You will improve very quickly.

3   Hold your maximum stretch for a count of 5, then slowly draw the leg back and place it in the starting position. Repeat the movement to the left and then perform the entire sequence twice.

Benefits
This movement is most beneficial for relieving stiffness and pain in the hip joint and for helping people with sciatica. It tones and firms the inner and outer thigh and releases tension in the lower back.

Stage two

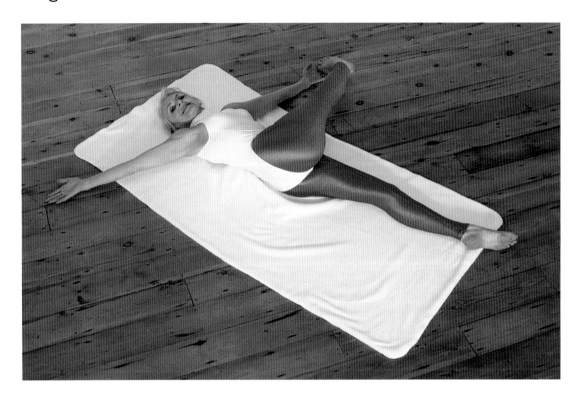

1 Lie flat on your back with your legs together, with your arms stretched out at shoulder level, palms uppermost.

2 Inhale deeply and, as you exhale, gently lift your right leg in the air. Keeping both legs straight, aim your right big toe to the centre of your left hand, but remember the halfway point is fine if your hip is stiff to start with.

3 Hold your maximum position for a count of 5, then inhale and carefully lift your right leg straight up in the air, then exhale as you slowly lower it back to its starting position. Repeat on the other side and then repeat the entire sequence twice.

Benefits
This movement is excellent for firming the midriff, waistline and abdominal muscles while sculpting the bottom and upper thighs. It is also excellent for relieving stiffness and pain in the hip and releasing tension in the lower back.

121

Stage three

1 Lie flat on your back with your arms straight, stretched back on the floor behind your head, and your legs straight and together.

2 Take a deep breath in and, as you exhale, lift your right leg in the air. Slowly lift your upper body and try to take hold of your right leg, ensuring that it remains straight. Your aim is to clasp your right big toe and aim the right knee to the right nostril. However, this is rarely possible at first, so clasp the leg wherever you can with ease and gently draw the leg towards the head. Ensure that both legs remain straight.

3 Hold the clasp for a count of 5, then slowly lower both the arms and leg back to their starting position and relax. Repeat this movement to the other side and then repeat the entire sequence twice.

Benefits
This movement stretches the hamstrings and tones and firms the front and back of the legs. It is also a brilliant abdominal firmer and toner. It relieves tension in the lower back and can be beneficial to those suffering from sciatica.

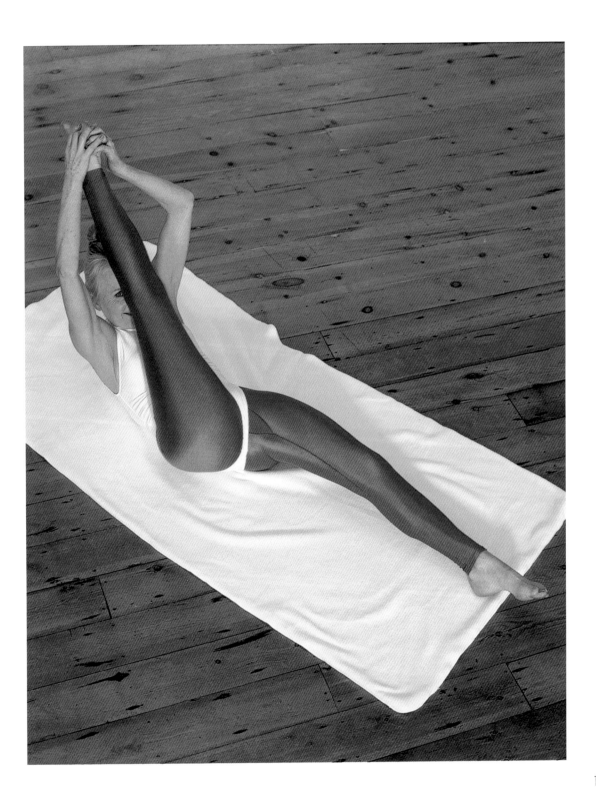

10 Crescent Moon

This is a beautiful backwards bend to firm your throat and thighs, and give your spine amazing flexibility.

Stage one

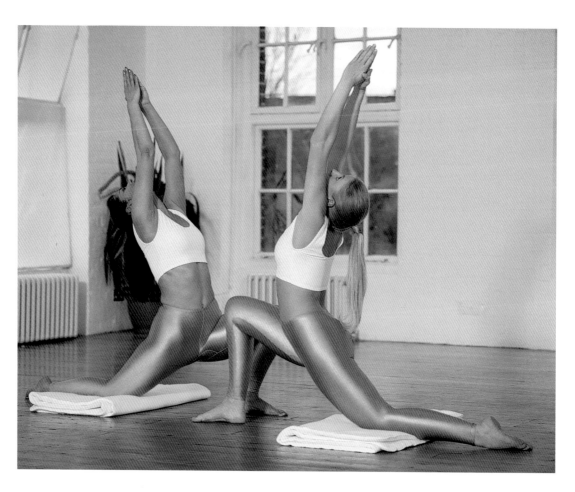

Make sure that you have a thick mat under your knees. Adopt a high kneeling position and place your right foot flat on the floor about 3 feet in front of your left knee, but in line with your right hip. Place both hands on your right knee then push your right buttock forwards, aiming the right buttock towards the right heel so stretching out the left leg. The front of the left calf should now be flat on the floor.

Lift both your arms in the air, placing your palms together. Inhale deeply and stretch your arms up above your head, dropping your head back and pointing your hands to the ceiling, keeping your eyes on your thumbs. Exhale and, breathing normally, hold this position for a count of 5, then inhale, lower your arms, exhale and relax. Repeat to the other side.

Stage two

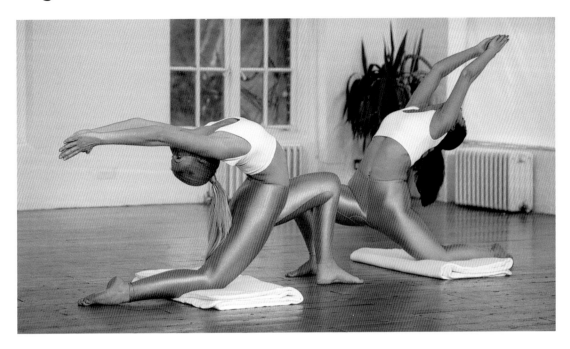

Only try this when you can accomplish Stage one without strain. Starting with your arms straight up in the air, as with Stage one, inhale and then slowly and carefully arch backwards.

Keep your lower body still and your arms straight, again keeping your eyes on your thumbs. Don't worry if you can only move back an inch at first. Just keep on practising and you will be delighted with your progress.

Breathing normally, hold your maximum position for a count of 5, increasing to a count of 10 as you progress. Inhale as you carefully return to an upright position.

Exhale, relax and repeat the movement on the other side. Repeat the entire sequence once.

Benefits
The Crescent Moon does wonders for your thighs – you can almost feel the cellulite disappearing. It relieves tension in your chest, gives your spine amazing flexibility, stimulates your kidneys and adrenal glands, tones and firms the jaw line and trims your waistline. It also gives you a beautiful warm glow of relaxed energy.

11 The Wheel

Please do not attempt if you are pregnant

Yoga's ultimate backwards stretch. This does wonders for your spine, your energy levels and your self-confidence, and it is just great to be able to do it – regardless of your age. Most of us can remember doing this as children, but after a gap – maybe a long gap – it takes a while to regain the necessary flexibility. It is best to do the movement in three stages.

Stage one

Lie flat on your back and draw your feet up to your body so that with your feet flat on the floor, your fingertips can just touch your feet. Your feet should be about 1 foot apart.

Place your arms by your sides. Inhale and, as you exhale, slowly lift your bottom from the floor. Tighten your abdominal muscles and your buttocks in this position, hold for a count of 5, then slowly lower your bottom to the floor. Relax and repeat 3 times.

Stage two

Lie flat on your back with your feet and arms as in Stage one.

This time, inhale and lift both your bottom and back from the floor so that only your feet, arms, head and shoulders remain on the floor.

Exhale again, tighten the buttocks and abdominal muscles, and hold for a count of 5. Then relax and repeat twice.

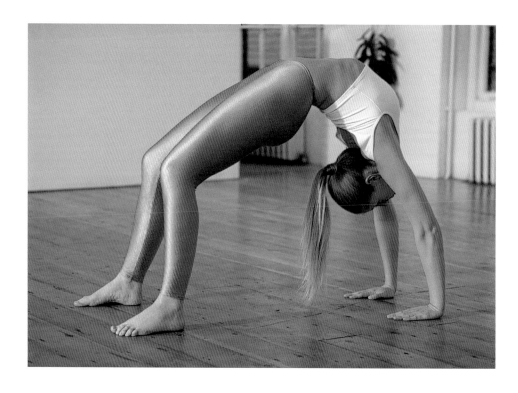

When you feel comfortable with the first two stages, then it is time to try the Wheel.

Stage three

Lie flat on your back with your feet about 1 foot apart and stretch your arms by your sides, your fingertips just touching your heels.

Then place your hands at shoulder level with your fingers pointing towards your feet. Check if this feels comfortable – sometimes it is not at all easy due to stiffness in the wrists and shoulders. If this is the case, wait until you are able to position your arms comfortably in this way before you progress. Now, with your feet and hands in the correct position, take a deep breath and, pushing down with the hands, aim to lift the entire body off the floor. It may take many attempts before you get much lift off, but with

practice it will happen – I promise! Once you are in your maximum position, exhale and hold, just for a second to begin with, increasing gradually until you are able to hold for a count of 10. Breathe normally in the maximum position. Aim eventually to straighten both your arms and legs in the maximum position.

Gently lower yourself to the floor and relax. Well done, your youth has returned!

Now draw your knees to your chest and rock from side to side and have a well-earned rest. Do not repeat this movement until you can do it easily – then do it twice.

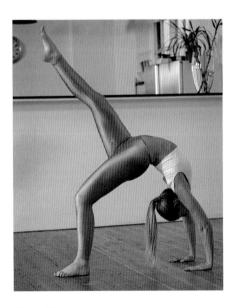

Stage four

Only try Stage four when you feel totally comfortable with your Wheel. In the Wheel, transfer your main body weight to your hands and try to lift a leg. Well done!

Then slowly release and lower your body to the floor. Draw your knees to your chest and gently rock your back from side to side.

Benefits
Energy and vitality normally decrease as the years advance. Also, the spine has a tendency to shorten and is frequently subject to degeneration in later years. The Wheel and the other yoga backwards bends will help to counteract this process. This movement stimulates extra blood to the spinal nerves, and tones and firms the arms, legs and abdominals.

My pupils in their 60s or 70s who manage to do it for the first time are absolutely delighted. It gives them tremendous confidence and it opens new horizons for them. They wonder that since they have accomplished this movement, what else is possible?

12   The Shoulderstand

This movement, the 'Mother of all Yoga Exercises', is regarded as the second most important posture in yoga – the most important being the Headstand.

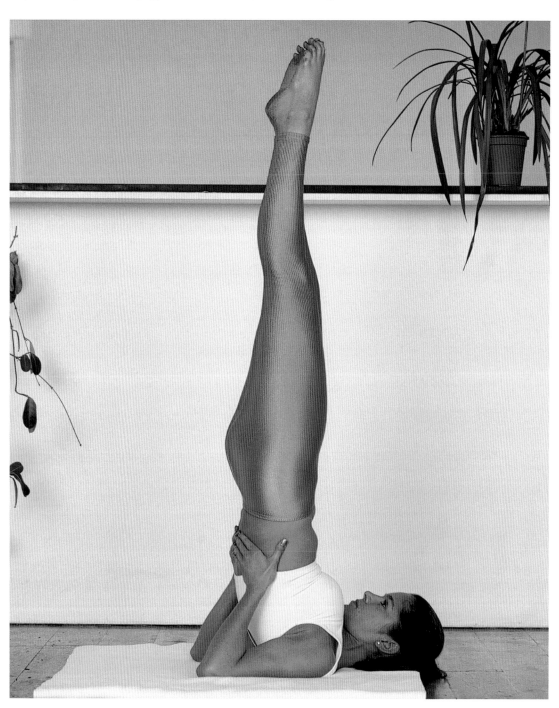

1 Lie flat on your back with your hands relaxed by your sides. Inhale deeply and, as you exhale, gently bend your knees and lift your feet, knees and buttocks off the floor. To support your back, place your hands at your waistline.

2 Keep lifting your legs until you reach your maximum position. Your eventual aim is to have your body in a perfect straight line. This might take you quite a while to achieve, but you will still be benefiting in the early stages of the movement.

Breathing normally, hold the movement for 30 seconds to begin with, gradually increasing by 30 seconds a week until you are able to hold for 3 minutes.

To come out of the posture, draw your knees to your forehead and then gently roll down your back, one vertebra at a time, until your bottom touches the floor. Then interlock your hands around your knees and rock slowly from left to right. Let your legs go straight out in front of you and relax. Follow with the Pose of a Fish. Relax for 5 minutes and do not repeat.

Benefits
This movement is so highly regarded because of its wonderful benefits to the entire body. It stimulates blood flow to the thyroid and parathyroid glands in the neck and it can assist a sluggish metabolism. It is a very soothing and energizing posture, helping to reverse the adverse ageing effects caused by gravity. It benefits the skin, hair and brain cells by stimulating extra blood flow to the head and neck areas. It strengthens the back, legs and abdominal muscles, and is beneficial for sufferers of varicose veins and haemorrhoids.

The extra blood flow to the chest can help people who suffer from chesty complaints such as asthma and bronchitis, and the extra blood flow to the head can help headache sufferers.

Shoulderstand
and the Bridge

From a beautifully straight Shoulderstand, ensure your hands are at your waistline and are supporting your lower body.

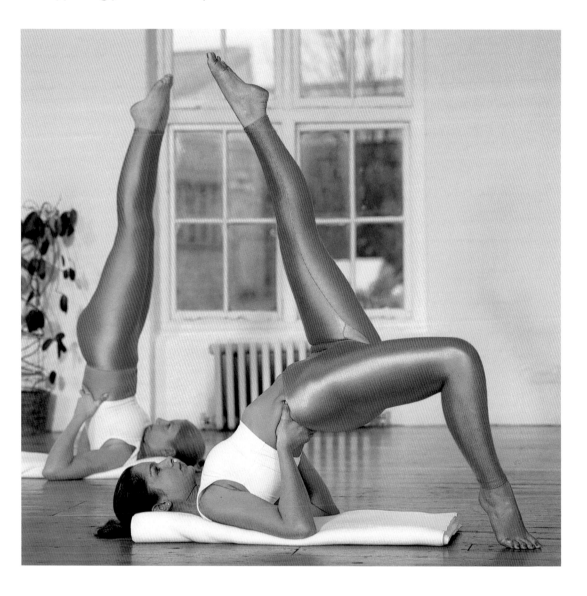

Try to drop one foot to the floor in front of your buttocks. This sounds easy, but it may take several attempts. As soon as one foot is resting comfortably on the floor, then try to take the other foot down and balance in the Bridge Position.

Hold this position for 10 seconds, then try to lift your legs up again one at a time into a perfect Shoulderstand. This may be difficult to start with so don't strain, but if you find it difficult in the beginning stages, then gently lower your body to the floor, lie down and relax. Eventually you will be able to manage the movement on both sides.

Come out of the movement exactly as you would for the Shoulderstand (see page 128) and finish the movement with the Pose of a Fish (see page 99).

Benefits
As well as all the benefits of the Shoulderstand, this movement greatly increases the strength and flexibility of the spine. When you have completed the variations on the Shoulderstand, then perform them in the following order to make a lovely Shoulderstand cycle.

○ *Shoulderstand*
○ *Balanced Shoulderstand*
○ *Shoulderstand and Bridge*
○ *Pose of Tranquillity*
○ *Pose of Tranquillity in Lotus Position*
○ *Pose of a Fish in Lotus Position.*

Talk about fit, flexible and fantastic. If you have completed this cycle, you are all of the above. Congratulations!

14 Pose of Tranquillity

Please do not attempt if you have high blood pressure

Please do not attempt if you are pregnant

Please do not attempt if you have head or neck problems

This movement can also be done from the Full Lotus Position, but should only be attempted when you are able to do the Full Lotus Position with comfort and ease.

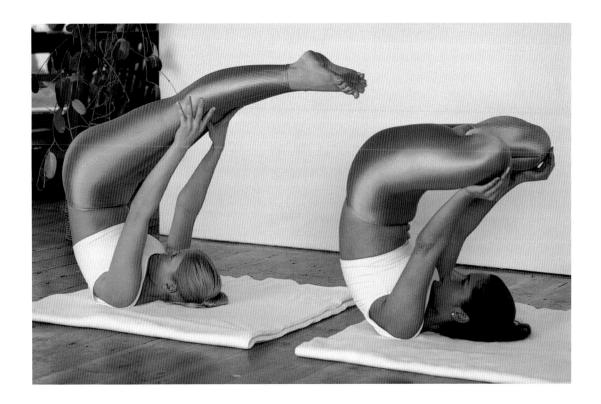

1 From the Shoulderstand, carefully lift your arms in the air and place them on your knees. The knees must be straight and as high as possible. Begin with trying this position with your legs together and then with your legs wide apart. Don't worry if you find balancing in this movement difficult at first. This is normal and with practice you will soon be able to do it.

Breathing normally, hold your position for a count of 30, increasing gradually until you are able to hold for 3 minutes.

2 Sit on your mat in the Full Lotus Position (see page 80). Gently lift your lower body from the floor and place your hands at your waistline to support your body.

Lift your legs as high as possible, still keeping them in the Lotus Position. When in your maximum position, balance and take your hands to your knees. Don't worry if you need to make several attempts before you achieve this. Hold the position for a count of 10 to start with, increasing slowly until you are able to hold for 3 minutes.

To come out of this position, move your hands back to your waistline, then gently start to lower your bottom to the floor, rolling down your spine very slowly, vertebra by vertebra, until your entire body is lying flat on the floor, but with your legs still entwined in the Lotus Position. Then move into the Lotus in Fish Position as follows.

Benefits
As well as all the benefits of the Shoulderstand, the Pose of Tranquillity is a balance and so it helps your coordination and balance. It is also incredibly soothing after a long busy day and is a wonderful tonic. This movement will really revive you, putting the sparkle back in your eyes and the roses in your cheeks.

15   Lotus in Fish Pose

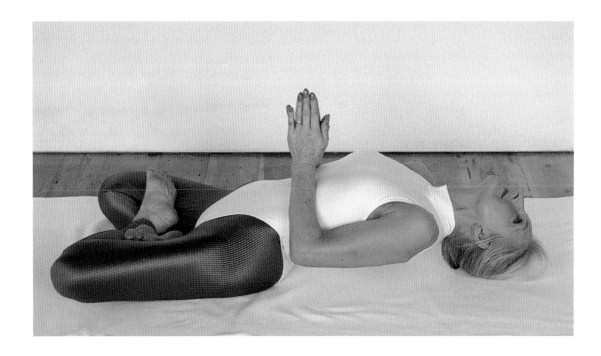

Bring the top of your head on to the floor, with your hands placed under your buttocks, thumbs touching, so that your upper body is supported by your elbows, and with your legs still in the Lotus Position.

Place your hands in prayer on your chest and rest in this position, breathing slowly and deeply for a count of 10.

Carefully lower your body to the floor and relax. Well done!

Benefits

The combination of the Pose of Tranquillity in Lotus Position and the Fish in Lotus Pose have all the benefits of the Shoulderstand, but they also keep the hips, knees and ankles incredibly flexible. In the Fish in Lotus Pose, the chest is expanded and deep breathing is made much easier. It is an excellent help for asthma sufferers. The thyroid and parathyroid glands in the neck receive a rich blood flow to them. Increased flexibility occurs in the spine, especially in the neck and lower back. It is a wonderful movement for toning and firming the muscles of the throat and jaw and for correcting poor posture.

16 The Classical Headstand

Please do not attempt if you have high blood pressure

Please do not attempt if you are pregnant

Please do not attempt if you have head or neck problems

This is the 'Father of all Yoga Exercises' and is a wonderful movement for the whole body. However, please do not attempt it until you have worked through and feel confident with the other movements in this book. By then your body will be sufficiently strong and flexible for you to be able to do it with ease. In the beginning stages it is wise to practise the movement by a wall to prevent you from falling.

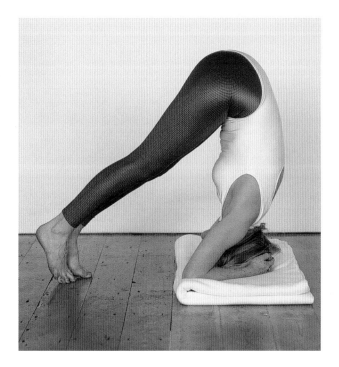

1 Fold your blanket into a thick cushion and, kneeling by your blanket, interlock your hands together to make a triangle. Place the triangle on the ground in front of you. Now lift one hand and touch your fingers to the centre of your other elbow then interlock your hands again. This ensures that your elbows are the right distance apart and the triangle you have made is exactly the right size for you. Now place the top of your head on the mat so that it is framed by your interlocked hands. Lift your bottom in the air and walk your feet towards your head. When you have reached your maximum position, hold it for a count of 5 then kneel down, keep your head down for a count of 10, then relax. Practise this small movement every day for two or three weeks before trying to progress any further. By doing this you will greatly strengthen your neck as well as accustoming your head to the extra blood flow. This ensures that everything is much easier when you come to do the Headstand.

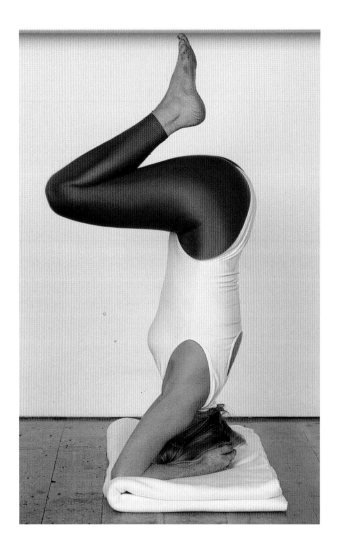

2 After repeating the preliminary stage, you will find that it seems your feet actually feel like leaving the floor, so now allow them to leave the floor and come into a crouching position. Stay in this balance for a few seconds and then straighten your legs into the Classical Headstand. Stay there for just a few seconds to begin with, increasing slowly as you become more confident in the movement until you are holding for 2 minutes.

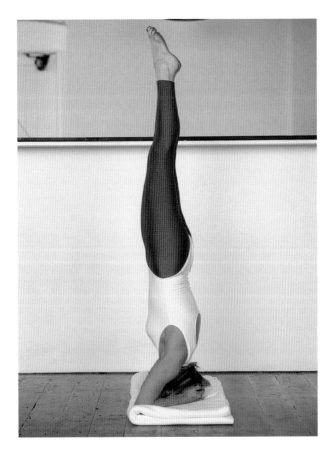

3 To come out of the movement, bend your knees back into a crouching position, and then come down very slowly, keeping your legs together until your feet touch the floor and then lower your bottom to your heels and relax.

Remain with your head down for a count of 10, allowing your circulation to return to normal. Then slowly return to a kneeling position. Well done!

Benefits
The benefits of this movement are huge. It is really invigorating and refreshing, and excellent for the brain, skin and hair. It can also help your eyesight, hearing and memory. The Hatha Yoga Pradipika states, 'On the first day he should remain only a little while in the headstand with legs in the air. This is viparitakarani. Increase the practice time a little each day. After six months grey hair and wrinkles completely disappear.' The headstand is one of Yoga's elixirs and helps to prevent the adverse ageing effects of gravity. Blood flow is stimulated to the pituitary gland and the pineal body, helping to keep these two glands in good condition.

17 Headstand in Pagoda

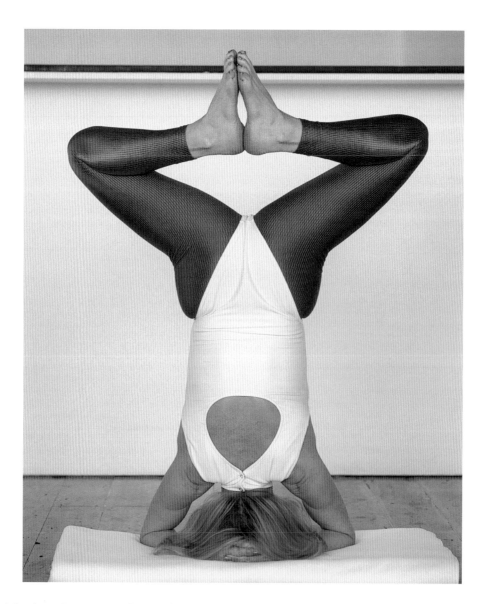

In the Headstand, open your legs wide and place your feet together in the middle. Then gently rotate your lower body to the right and then to the left.

Benefits
This is excellent for your flexibility, balance and coordination.

18 Headstand in the Half Split

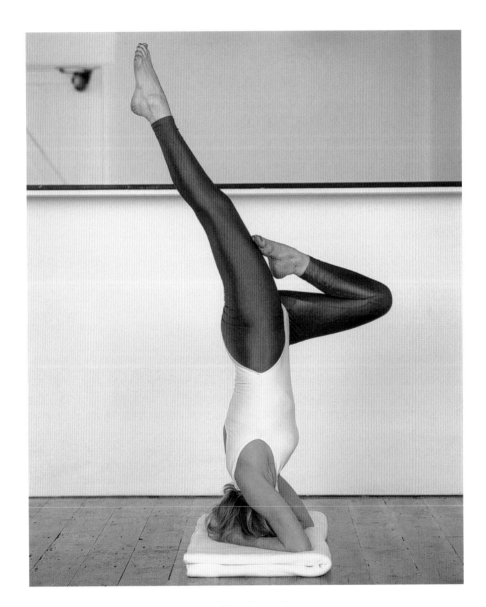

In the Headstand, gently slide one foot down the opposite thigh. Hold and repeat to the other side.

Benefits
This is excellent for your concentration, balance and flexibility.

139

19 Headstand in Full Lotus

Please do not attempt if you have high blood pressure

Please do not attempt if you are pregnant

Please do not attempt if you have head or neck problems

Achieving this movement could take a while – it took me ages but I was ecstatic when I finally managed it, so please don't give up. It is only possible when your joints are sufficiently flexible to do the Full Lotus Position with ease.

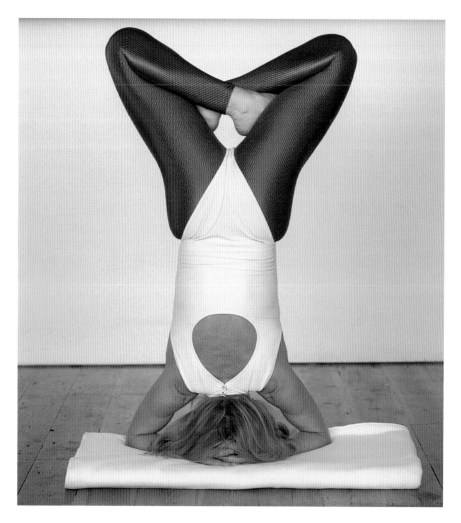

In the Headstand, place your right foot on your left thigh and then your left foot on your right thigh to assume the Full Lotus Position.

Hold the position for a count of 10, then undo your legs and repeat the movement the other way round.

Benefits
This gives you amazing coordination, balance and flexibility.

20 The Plough with Extra Movements

We first started the Plough in the previous chapter, 'Power Stretching' (see page 97). Now that you have progressed to the advanced class you might like to progress to the next stages and learn some more movements in this position.

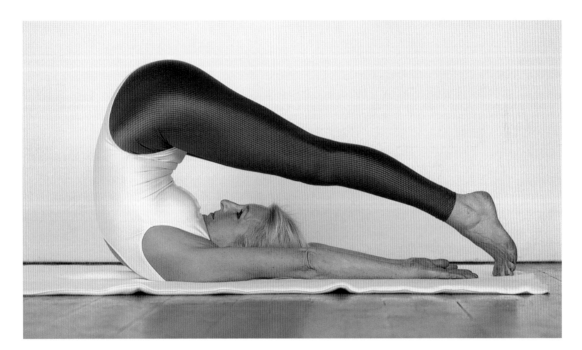

1 Lie flat on your back, bend your knees and gently lift your bottom off the floor into the Plough position.

2 Hold this position and then allow your legs to stretch out to the floor, interlocking your hands behind your back.

3 Once Stage two has become comfortable, unclasp your hands and stretch them towards your feet for a stretch to your shoulders.

Benefits
This is excellent for releasing shoulder tension.

21 Wide-angled Plough

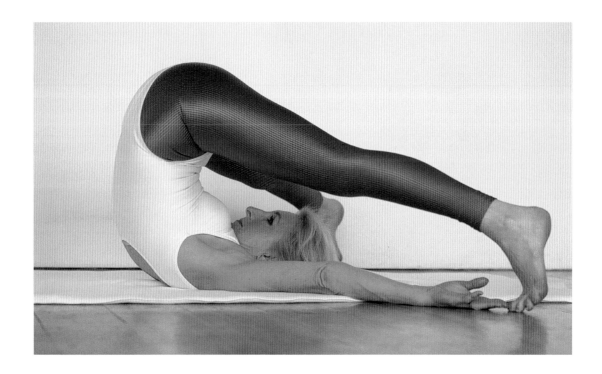

Once Stage three of the Plough becomes comfortable, then open your legs wide in the movement and stretch your hands towards your wide-open legs.

Benefits
This gives extra flexibility to your hips.

22 The Noose Pose

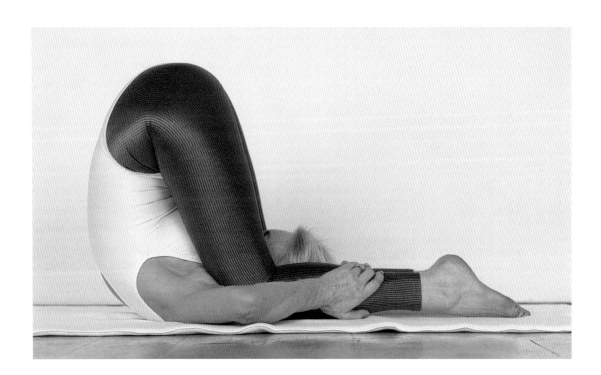

In your normal Plough position, gently draw your knees by your ears and place your hands on your calves.

Benefits
This lovely position greatly increases the flexibility of your lower back.

143

23 The Sleeping Pose

Only try this when you are fully flexible and comfortable in the Noose Pose.

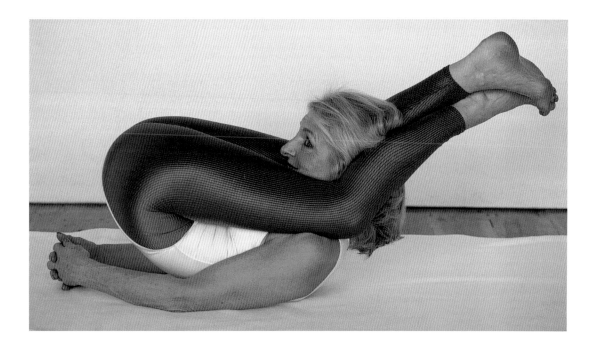

In the Noose Pose, cross your ankles, hold your calves and carefully try to lift your head between your legs. This is a very strong movement, so don't strain. It will happen when you are ready.

To come out of the position, uncross your ankles, draw your knees to your forehead and roll down your back, one vertebra at a time, until you are lying flat on the floor. Breathe in, place your hands under your buttocks and arch your back into the Pose of a Fish (see page 99). Lie flat and relax. Now draw your knees to your chest and rock your back gently from side to side, then lie down and relax your entire body.

Benefits
Along with all the benefits of the Plough, this incredible movement is wonderful for increasing flexibility of the neck and shoulders, lower back and hips and, believe it or not, when you get there it is comfortable.

24 Deep Relaxation

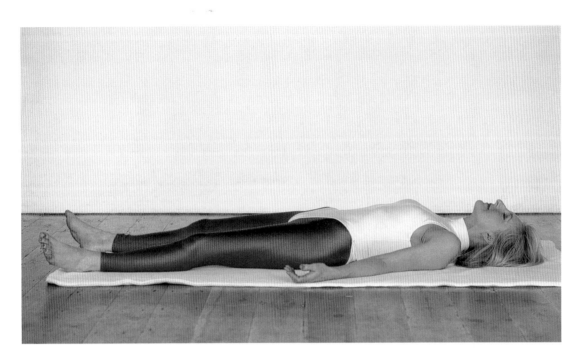

Lie flat on your back with your legs 2 feet apart, arms 1 foot from your body, and relax your ankles and feet, relax your calves and thighs and feel your legs becoming really relaxed.

With your palms uppermost, relax your back and shoulders. Keep your breathing slow and deep, concentrating on the slow calm exhalation. Roll your eyeballs upwards, let your scalp slide back, smooth out all your facial muscles and let your body relax into a lovely dreamy and drowsy state.

Imagine you are floating on a beautiful warm ocean with nothing but beautiful clear blue sky up above you. Float on and on and on in the ocean. Keep this in your mind, relax, relax, relax. Stay relaxed for 5–10 minutes, then take a deep breath and visualize fresh vitalizing energy flowing through your body.

The cure for all the illness of life is stored in the inner depth of life itself. The access to which becomes possible when we are alone. This solitude is a world in itself, full of wonders and resources unthought of. It is absurdly near, yet so unapproachably distant.

RABINDRANATH TAGORE

Salute to the Sun

 Straight Leg Triangle

 Standing Head to Knee Posture

 Pose of a Tree

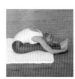 Pose of a Sage

 Back Stretch

 Pose of a Bow

 Pose of a Tortoise

 Maltese Cross

Crescent Moon

 The Wheel

 The Shoulderstand

 Shoulderstand and the Bridge

 Pose of Tranquillity

Lotus in Fish Pose

 The Classical Headstand

 Headstand in Pagoda

 Headstand in the Half Split

 Headstand in Full Lotus

 The Plough with Extra Movements

 Wide-angled Plough

 The Noose Pose

 The Sleeping Pose

 Deep Relaxation

10-MINUTE YOGA WORKOUTS

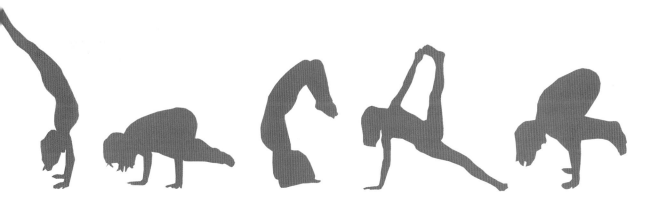

the yoga hand balances

I am now going to show you eight yoga hand balances. These movements are powerful strengtheners and toners for the arms. It is not easy to teach these balances because people tend to have a lot of weakness in the wrists, and the arms must be gradually strengthened until they are able to support the body's weight. Yoga movements that involve the arms bearing the body's weight, strengthen the arms carefully and thoroughly. My pupils are thrilled at the wonderful tone and shape that the hand balances give to their arms and shoulders.

Only try one balance a day and no more, otherwise you run the risk of straining your arms. If you have recently had any injury to your arms, wrists or shoulders, make sure that you are fully recovered before you start to practise the movements. Then progress very gently, limiting the holds to a count of 1 in the beginning stages.

chapter nine

1 Pose of a Crow

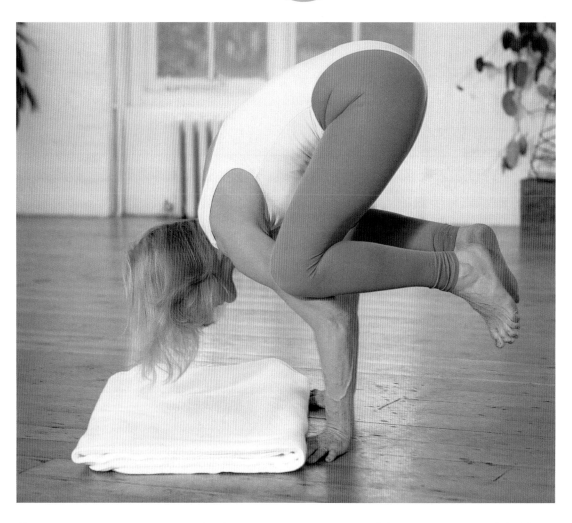

Come into a squatting position and make sure you have a folded blanket in front of you in case you topple over in your first attempts. Spread your hands out with your fingers wide apart and position them comfortably in front of you.

Choose a spot and concentrate hard on it, inhale deeply and, resting your knees on the outer portion of the upper arms, carefully lift your legs from the floor keeping your head up.

This is difficult at first, but you will have a great feeling of achievement once you have managed it. Hold for a count of 5, increasing to 10 as you progress, then come out of it calmly and slowly. Repeat once.

Benefits
It strengthens the shoulders, arms and wrists, expands the chest and strengthens your powers of concentration.

2 Pose of a Raven

Please do not attempt if you are pregnant

Make sure you have padding on the floor in front of you in case you topple over during your first attempts.

Again, this takes practice and amazing concentration, but you'll make it.

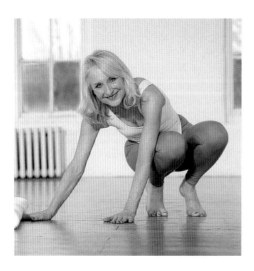

1 Squat and place both arms to the right of your body with your hands about 1 foot apart.

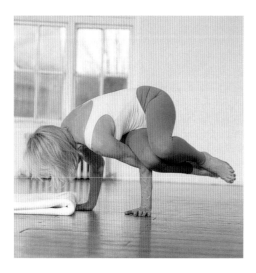

2 Inhale and bend your elbows and, keeping your head up as you exhale, place both knees on the left upper arm. Concentrate on a spot to help you balance and lift your legs from the floor.

Hold for a count of 3 to start with, increasing to 10 as you progress. Come out of the movement slowly and repeat on the other side. Do not repeat.

Benefits
This is excellent for strengthening the wrists and arms. It tones the lower abdomen and is great for your patience and concentration.

3 Sideways Body Raise
(Advanced Position)

Please do not attempt if you are pregnant

We first practised the Sideways Body Raise in Chapter 6 (see page 66). This will have greatly strengthened your arms, so it will be exciting to try this slightly stronger stage of the movement. Go carefully and remember, don't strain.

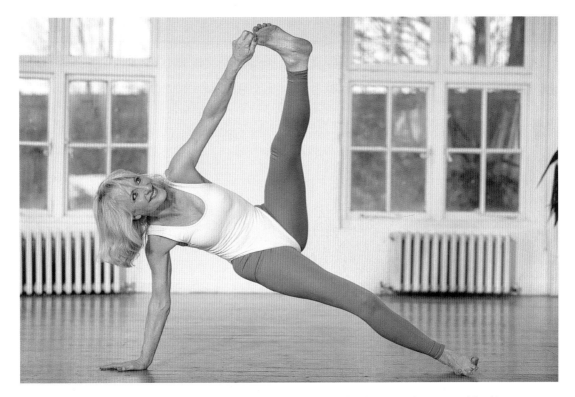

In the Full Sideways Body Raise, bring the arm that is alongside your ear on the floor in front of you in line with your hips.

Now place your upper foot next to this hand and, staring at a spot to help your balance, grasp your big toe and lift the leg, straightening the arm and leg. When fully balanced, turn your

head and look upwards at your lifted leg. Hold for a count of 5, increasing to 10 as you progress.

Gently lower your head, relocating a spot on the floor to help you balance, then gently lower your body to the floor, relax and repeat on the other side. Do not repeat the whole movement.

Benefits
This movement tones and firms the arms, wrists and shoulders and greatly increases the flexibility of your lower back and hip area. It is also wonderful for your patience and concentration.

4   Pose of a Peacock

Please do not attempt if you are pregnant

I think this is my favourite balance. It gives me an amazing feeling of energy.
This is not easy, but keep practising and it will happen. You will be thrilled when it does.

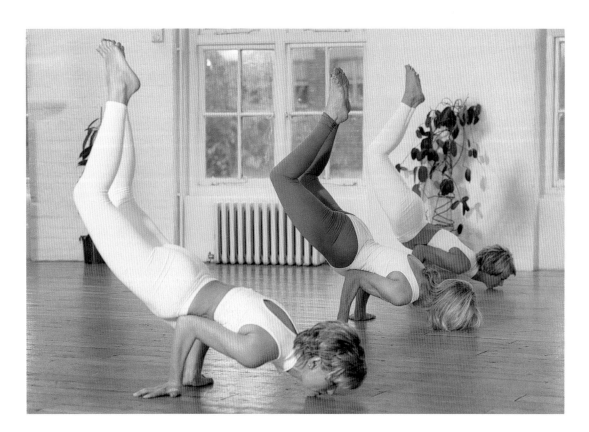

Kneel and place your hands on the floor as close as possible together, with your fingers out to the sides or backwards. (Some of my students prefer one method and some the other.)

Bring your body forward so you feel your elbows on the inside of your hip bones. Now aim to lift your legs from the floor and hold for a count of 5, then slowly lower your legs to the floor and relax.

For the advanced pose, place your chin on the floor and lift your legs higher. Again, hold for 5 at first, increasing to 10 as you progress.

Benefits
Again, this movement greatly strengthens the arms, wrists and concentration. It also massages the digestive organs and pancreas and can be beneficial for diabetics. It can also help relieve constipation and indigestion. The Pose of a Peacock can do wonders for your self-confidence – once you manage it, you realize the huge potential that is there inside you!

5 Pose of an Elephant

Please do not attempt if you are pregnant

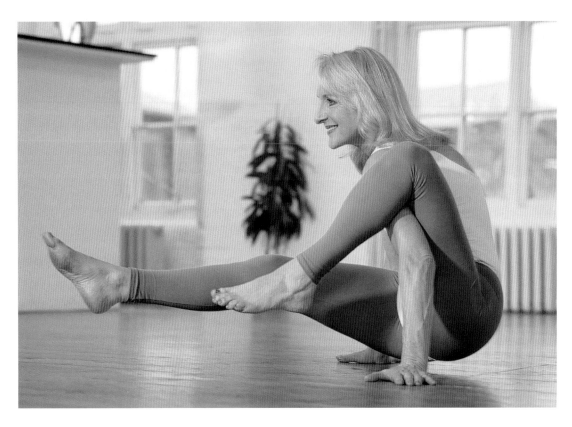

Sit straight with both legs straight out in front of you with your hands on the floor beside you.

Leaning forward, place your right leg over your right upper arm. Keep your left leg straight. Place your hands beside your hips with your fingers pointing forward. Take a deep breath and as you exhale leaning forward, balancing on your hands, lift your bottom and left leg from the floor, ensuring that your left leg stays straight.

Hold for a count of 3 to start with, increasing to 5 as you progress. Gently lower yourself to the floor, relax and then repeat to the other side. Do not repeat the movement.

Benefits
This tones and strengthens the arms, wrists and shoulders. It is also a very powerful toner for the upper thighs.

6   Pose of a Firefly

Please do not attempt if you are pregnant

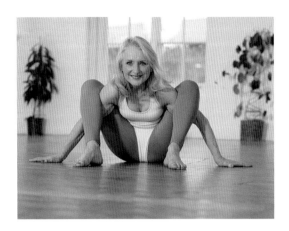

1 Sit down with both legs straight out in front of you. Bend your legs so that your feet and knees are about 1 foot apart. Inhale and place your hands in prayer, then lower your elbows towards the floor between your knees and stretch out your hands so that your hands and elbows are on the outer side of the knee. If you cannot yet manage to have your elbows on the outside of the knee, then practise until you can before you attempt this movement.

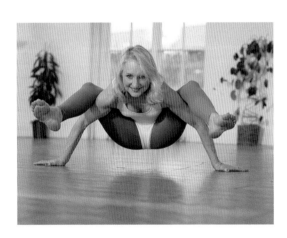

2 Stretch your arms back a little and then, leaning slightly forward, gently lift your bottom and legs from the floor, balancing on your hands. Breathing normally, hold for a count of 5, then gently lower your bottom to the floor and relax. Repeat once.

Benefits
This is a wonderful toner and strengthener for the shoulders, wrists and arms. This movement also increases the flexibility of your lower back and hips.

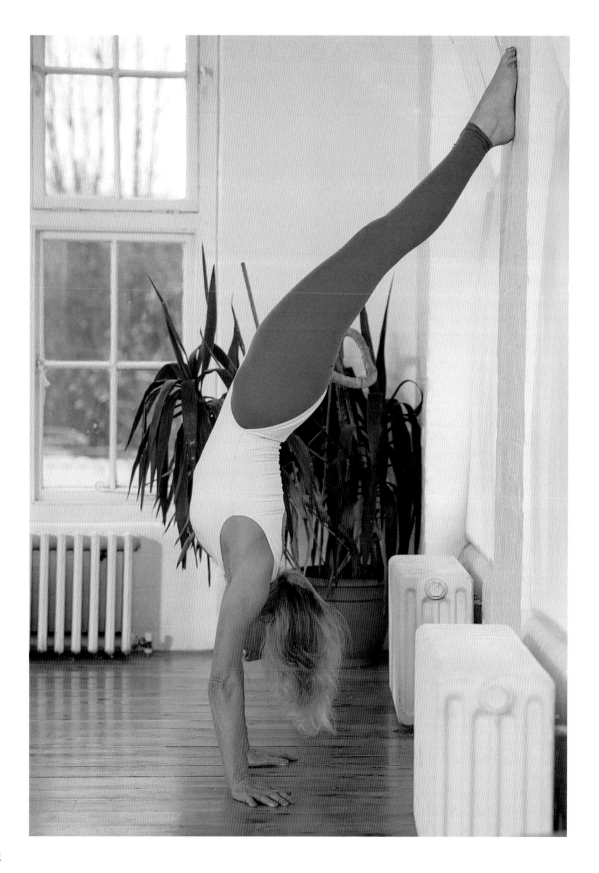

7　Handstand

Please do not attempt if you have high blood pressure

Please do not attempt if you are pregnant

So many of my students gasp when they see this pose for the first time. They regard it as a relic of their childhood and are amazed at its incredible energizing benefits, once they have re-learnt the movement.

Stand straight and place your hands flat on the floor, shoulder width apart and about 1 foot away from a wall. Make sure your arms are straight.

Inhale and, as you exhale, aim to lift your legs and swing them up to the wall. Don't worry if the first time you attempt this movement it just resembles a small jump. Just keep practising and gradually that energy and flexibility will return.

Once you can manage it with ease, take your feet away from the wall and aim to balance with your toes pointed and head raised.

Hold for a count of 5 to begin with, increasing to 10 as you progress. Once you are able to balance with ease, try the movement away from the wall. Make sure that you have a couple of friends to catch you if necessary until you are confident in the movement.

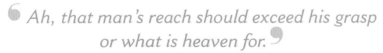

❛ Ah, that man's reach should exceed his grasp or what is heaven for. ❜
ROBERT BROWNING, from *Andrea del Sarto*

Benefits
As well as strengthening the arms, shoulders and wrists, the Handstand expands the chest and is excellent for the skin, hair and brain cells due to the increased blood flow to that area. This pose makes me feel great – I feel like a teenager again!

8 Pose of a Scorpion

This is a wonderful movement. My pupils think that they will never manage it but, when they do, it gives them such confidence.

Note that it is possible to do this posture from a Headstand once your Headstand is stable. However, to begin with I prefer to start pupils by a wall, with me by their side to watch, steady and encourage them.

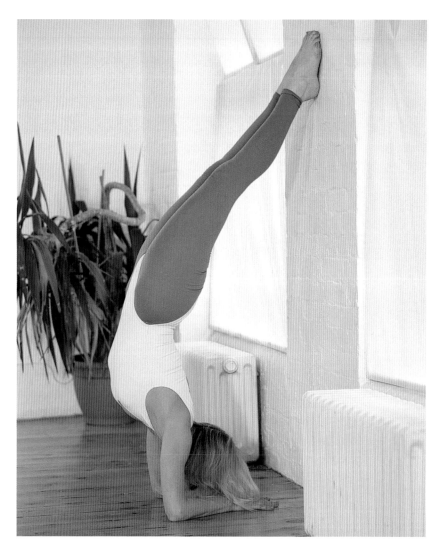

1 Place a non-slip mat by a wall and kneel on it. Place you hands and elbows on your mat, shoulder width apart with your thumbs pointing towards each other. Keep your head up. Now lift your bottom in the air, straighten your legs and walk your feet towards your elbows.

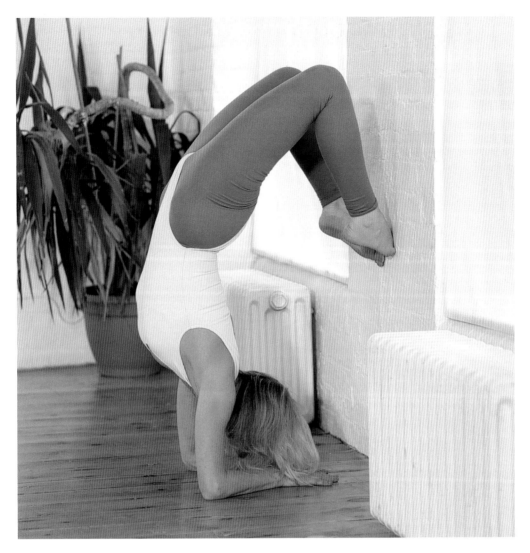

2 Inhale and, as you exhale, kick your legs upwards, aiming your feet to touch the wall, ensuring that your head stays up and off the floor. This will take several attempts, but just keep trying. Once your feet are comfortably on the wall, then try to balance, taking your feet away from the wall just a few inches at first, aiming to hold for a count of 5. Once you can manage this with ease, then try walking your feet down the wall in the direction of your head. Breathing normally, hold for a count of 5, then gently come out of the position. Lower your bottom to your heels and relax in the Pose of a Swan and hold this movement for a count of 5, breathing normally.

Benefits
This pose is excellent for your balance and concentration and it is an amazing confidence booster. It removes tension from your shoulders and neck and it strengthens your arms, elbows and hands.

part three

Total Health with Yoga

yoga and diet

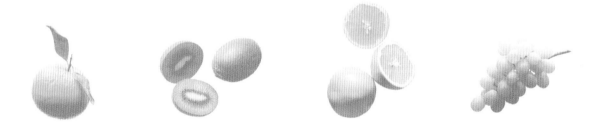

chapter ten

If you have already started practising the postures in this book, I hope you will have found that your flexibility is getting better, you have more energy, your shape is improving and you are finding it easier to cope with life's many challenges.

All these benefits and many others start to appear, sometimes as if out of the blue. Many subtle changes occur in your body and often this prompts people to question their diet. Once you start feeling good about yourself you stop wanting to harm your body; junk foods that you may have once referred to as 'treats' may not have the same appeal and eventually you will regard them as toxins. This is yoga's way of naturally encouraging you to eating foods that are beneficial to your body and that enhance the prana or life force within you.

As yoga continues to stimulate this flow of positive health within you, you will notice other changes happening. It is likely that your tastes will alter, you go off foods and drinks that you once thought you couldn't live without. You start to listen to your body. It is usual for my pupils to admit that before they took up yoga they would regularly enjoy a heavy meal washed down with two or three glasses of wine, but that nowadays their preference is for a lighter, fresher meal with one glass or none at all. This is the best and most natural way to lose weight and cultivate leanness, positive health and vitality.

The more you progress in yoga the more these changes are effected from within, but a lot of my pupils are keen to hurry things along. They see their shape changing due to the exercises and ask me for dietary advice. They want results now! This is why I set out below my own eating plan that has helped thousands of my students.

Over 40 years ago, as part of my nursing training, I had the good fortune to work on a ward specializing in nutritional and metabolic problems and eating disorders. This gave me a lifelong interest in nutrition. I realized that if we ate fresh, healthy foods in as natural a state as possible, our bodies would glow with positive health and well-being. I understood that whatever diet we choose, it must fit in with our lifestyle and cope with our social and work commitments. Also, it must be well balanced to give us all the nutrients we need to keep us slim and healthy and to provide us with energy.

I designed my plan when my own weight fluctuations and lack of energy made me listen to the experts with whom I was working. Over the years, I have adapted the plan to fit in with changes in my own life, as well as integrating the knowledge I have since gained about yoga and nutrition. However, the basic plan is still very much the same – simple, fresh, healthy food in the correct quantities to maintain our weight easily and effortlessly, and, most importantly, to keep us healthy and give us energy.

Back in the Stone Age, man's diet would have consisted of fresh fruits, vegetables, meat and fish. In those days there was no processed, tinned or packaged food, no fast food, and no quick 'heat and serve' meals. Early man had no insecticides, additives, preservatives or E numbers to contend with. This was all brought home to me when I presented doctors with the results of tests on my patients in the nutrition ward where I was working. In the ward there was one lady with a severe eating disorder and no treatment had been of help. I mentioned to the doctors that I had seen junk food and drink being smuggled to her by visiting relatives on many occasions – maybe this should be taken into consideration. One doctor suddenly said, 'Barbara, if we all ate simple food in as fresh and natural state as possible, so many of these problems and disorders could be eliminated.'

I will remember those words for the rest of my life because, until that moment, I had thought of my nutritional work as something only relating to my patients, but when I thought of my own health, everything seemed to click into place. So, I designed my fabulous natural food plan and reaped the wonderful benefits. I am glad that I learnt so young!

I am not going to list all the vitamins and their benefits – that information is available everywhere. But it is vital to understand that although tinned and frozen fruits and vegetables can be shown to have the same amount of vitamins as fresh produce, they lack the essence called prana or life force contained in fresh fruits and vegetables. This cannot be seen or measured but, believe me, it is there!

My Plan

RULES

○ Eat three meals a day and nothing in between apart from the recommended drinks.

○ Never eat standing up. Sit down and enjoy your food.

○ Make your food look beautiful, garnish it with herbs, have flowers on the table or light scented candles in the evening.

○ If you are out at a dinner party, don't offend your hosts by refusing their food. If an item is served that is not on your plan, then just accept a small portion. If you would like two glasses of wine during a special evening, then simply go without the previous evening.

○ If you are in a tremendous hurry and have no time for lunch or to prepare any of the items suggested, then:

a) have 2 bananas – they are excellent for lunch when you are in a rush and are the most perfectly packaged 'fast food', containing many essential vitamins and minerals;

b) when at home, place 1 small carton of natural organic yoghurt, 1 banana, 1 teaspoon of honey and 1 carton of raspberries in a blender and drink this for your lunch. This is fabulous – healthy, nutritious and delicious!

○ If one day you break your diet and eat some junk food, don't feel guilty and cut back the next day. Just accept the fact that you are human. Start back on the plan the next day.

[Note: I advise you to consult your doctor or nutritionist before starting on this or any other eating plan to make sure that it is suitable for your personal dietary requirements.]

PERMITTED FOODS

Fresh Fruit
One portion equals one of each of the following:

apple	½ small melon
pear	large slice of water melon
orange	½ grapefruit
peach	3 apricots
small banana	3 plums
dish of berries	3 figs

These are only examples. All fresh fruit is allowed. Do not use tinned, frozen or stewed fruit.

Fresh vegetables and salads
All vegetables are allowed except crisps, chips, potatoes and corn on the cob. The latter two may be eaten occasionally as a substitute for rice and pasta for dinner. Try to have as much variety as possible. Have them raw, steamed, boiled or stir-fried – never deep-fried.

1 portion = 3 tablespoons of cooked vegetables.

Salad Ingredients
Have as much as you like but make sure the ingredients are fresh and raw. Only use 1 tablespoonful of dressing.

Fish
All varieties are allowed. Grill, steam, poach or pan fry with very little oil. Do not deep fry. Try to have oily fish 3 times a week.

Chicken, poultry, game and veal
All varieties are allowed. Grill, poach, steam, barbecue – do not deep fry.

Red meat
Beef, lamb, pork, venison, etc. Have no more than twice a week.

Eggs and cheese
Both are allowed in the amounts shown.

Grains
Only whole grains are allowed and in the amounts shown. No white bread, rice or pasta.

Milk
Semi-skimmed (½ pint daily) and natural yoghurt in the amounts indicated.

Not permitted – until you have reached your desired weight

bagels	hot chocolate
beer	ice cream
biscuits	jam
breakfast cereals	puddings
buns	soft drinks
cakes	spirits
canned drinks	sugar
chips	sweets
chocolates	

Additives and preservatives
Avoid all additives and preservatives. Just eat natural healthy food.

BREAKFAST

Choose from:

1 portion fresh fruit and 1 natural yoghurt;

2 portions of any fresh fruit chopped up, drizzled with 1 teaspoon of honey;

1oz of sliced hard cheese or 4oz cottage cheese with 1 sliced apple or pear;

1 slice granary toast with a little butter and either 1 piece of fresh fruit or a glass of fresh fruit juice;

1 poached egg on a slice of granary toast with a scraping of butter.

plus
Tea or coffee from your allowance.

LUNCH

Choose from:

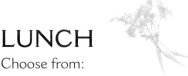

4oz chicken, turkey or fish; or 2 eggs, 2oz cheese; or 4oz red meat (remember, red meat is allowed only twice a week) with large salad — use a variety of raw fresh ingredients to make your choice different every day, together with 1 tablespoon olive oil and vinegar dressing. Instead of salad, you may have 2 fresh-cooked vegetables;

1 sandwich made with 2 slices wholegrain bread and a scraping of butter or mayonnaise, filled with salad and 2oz of chicken, turkey or fish, or 1 egg or 1oz cheese;

1/2 avocado pear filled with 3oz prawns, topped with 1 dessertspoon marie rose dressing or lemon mayonnaise and garnish with green salad;

1 Caesar salad using cos lettuce, 1 tablespoon dressing, 1 1/2 oz Parmesan cheese and 1/2 slice granary toast made into garlic croutons;

Salade Nicoise — lettuce, tomatoes, green beans (cooked), 5 black olives, 3oz tuna fish, and 1/2 hard-boiled egg, with 1 tablespoon oil and vinegar dressing.

DINNER

Choose from:

Starter

melon;

fresh asparagus with a little butter or vinaigrette;

clear soup;

tomato salad;

mixed salad;

mini Caesar salad (without croutons).

Main Course

4oz chicken, fish, veal or red meat (remember, red meat is allowed only twice a week);

small wholegrain, rice or pasta dish;

1 large bowl of mussels cooked in garlic, wine and onions;

large platter of mixed grilled seafood including prawns, salmon, langoustine and calamari;

plus

2 fresh vegetables or a large raw salad with 1 tablespoonful of oil and vinegar dressing.

Dessert

1 piece fresh fruit.

plus

Tea or coffee from your allowance.

To drink

6–8 glasses of water a day;

herbal tea as desired;

coffee and tea, preferably decaffeinated, no more than 5 cups a day;

wine – 1 glass a day, with dinner if desired.

Copy this plan, slip it in your bag and take it everywhere.

There is plenty of choice in the plan, so it will fit into the busiest lifestyle and cope with any social engagement, but it is important to vary your diet to make sure you have all the vitamins and minerals you require. For instance, if you have chicken with salad for lunch, then have fish and vegetables for dinner.

By keeping to this plan, it is easily possible to lose 2–3 lbs a week. Once you have reached your desired weight, gradually increase the amount you eat until you find how much you need to maintain this weight. If you gain another 3–4lbs, then immediately return to your plan until your weight is corrected. You will find that you gradually reach a level where your weight stays the same and you are able to maintain it effortlessly and naturally. Then you will keep in shape for life.

If you are happy with your weight and just want to eat for excellent health, then follow the plan and increase the amounts of the foods in accordance with your taste and appetite.

Finally, I am often asked if I am a vegetarian, as is the preference of many yoga devotees. I have tried a vegetarian diet but, quite honestly, it does not suit me and I feel much better for including meat, fish and chicken in my diet. The choice must be an individual one. Listen to your body and make a personal decision according to what feels right for you. Good luck and good health!

Men who are pure like food which is pure, which gives health, mental power, strength and long life, which has taste, is soothing and nourishing and which makes glad the heart of man.

BHAGAVAD GITA 17.8

meditation

chapter eleven

With our body disciplined and in great shape through practising yoga exercises and our health enhanced by eating fresh, vital foods, our physical being should now be in excellent condition. All that remains now is for our mind to become calm, alert and focused. In the West there is a tendency to resort to tranquillizers to calm the mind, caffeine and other toxic substances to stimulate energy, alcohol to help us relax and sleeping pills to aid sleep. When stress manifests as disease we visit the doctor and are prescribed pills to calm the condition that has been triggered by lack of attention to the body's warning signs. For over 5,000 years, techniques for stilling and calming the mind have been an integral part of yoga. Collectively, these are known as meditation.

Meditation is really very simple. When the mind is bombarded with thoughts, it is probably because it is concentrating on an anxiety about something in the future or a worry about the past. Meditation replaces these thought processes with something very simple such as concentrating on your breathing. You focus your mind in the present, giving your thought processes a well-deserved rest.

How to Meditate

- Sit in a comfortable position and make sure that you are warm – your body temperature can drop a little during meditation. The Lotus Position is perfect, but if you are not comfortable in this, then your favourite armchair will do just fine.
- Make sure that you will not be disturbed. Take your telephone off the hook and, if necessary, put a 'do not disturb' sign on your door.
- If you have an important appointment later in the day, make sure you set your alarm clock for the appropriate time. It is not unusual to fall asleep during your first attempts at meditation.
- Focus on an object. Choose something that works for you, such as a beautiful flower, a candle flame (make sure it is safe in case you fall asleep) or a religious symbol. Anything that works for you is fine. If no suitable object is on hand, then close your eyes and concentrate on your breathing.
- When your mind wanders away from your chosen object to your anxieties, worries or random thoughts, realize that this is normal and happens to most people. Just let your worries float past you and gently bring your mind back to your chosen object.

DON'T EXPECT MIRACLES

Meditation, like everything else in life, requires practise. Sometimes it is very difficult to switch off and at times like these we need to adopt a detached attitude and relax, realizing that this is the present moment just as it is. You will benefit from all your meditations, although some will be more relaxing than others. The relaxing effect will stay with you for quite a while so try to meditate for a number of short periods of time every day –

5 minutes is fine. You will find your overall stress levels reduce dramatically and your mind will become clear, calm, energized and focused.

As you progress, lengthen your meditations to 10–20 minutes. You will frequently receive new insights into a particular area of your life and, when the mind is peaceful and calm, you will often discover your way ahead to be much clearer. Time 'taken out' to meditate always pays for itself handsomely as after meditation you are much more productive than beforehand.

OTHER MEDITATION TECHNIQUES

Once you realize the necessity to switch off for a moment during your day, you can incorporate meditation into your daily life. For instance:

o   Sit in the garden and listen to bird song or just concentrate on a beautiful sky.
o   Some people find it easier to meditate if they repeat a word or phrase (this is known as a mantra). The constant repetition of a mantra can make it easier to switch off your thought processes, enabling the mind to calm. Choose a word that works for you; 'calm', 'peace' and 'love' are all fine, or you may use the yoga word 'om' (pronounced 'aum', it means 'what was, what is and what shall be'). Take a deep breath and, as you exhale, repeat 'om' slowly and calmly, over and over again. Yogis believe this to be the natural sound of the universe.
o   It can be great to meditate while exercising – the yoga balances are meditation in motion.

Once meditation becomes a part of your life, you will find it easy to switch into meditation mode during your day and you will learn to relax and focus your mind at odd moments. This way you will prevent the over-burdening effect of stress becoming a serious problem. By meditating, we are not trying to find peace and calm – they are already within us. We are trying to shut off the overload of mental stimuli, enabling us to give our natural peace a place in our hectic lives.

After you have been practising meditation for a while you will have the experience of a deeply relaxed thoughtless state. This is referred to as 'going into the gap'. The gap will gradually become easier to access and, by doing so, inner peace and silence will become a larger part of your life. In the gap, you establish contact with the universal spirit, the source of your own natural, unlimited, internal intelligence. Once you have put your trust in this you are guided from within and from there nothing is impossible. You experience a sense of beautiful inner joy and confidence.

Silence is the element in which great things fashion themselves together.

yoga and your
health problems

chapter twelve

When you take time out to practise yoga movements and deep breathing, meditate and eat healthy foods you will find that your overall health starts to improve dramatically. And as your health improves your health problems gradually lessen.

Having said this, I still find pupils who wish to learn an exercise to help with a particular health problem! Ill health is a manifestation of imbalance within the body and although there are movements that are extremely beneficial for specific problems, there can be no short cut.

Your body needs daily exercise and if your time is limited to the Ten-minute Miracle then that will do fine. You must also learn to relax during the day, even if you only take short breaks and totally relax in your office chair. Slow deep breathing can be fitted in to the busiest day and it is especially beneficial if taken in fresh air. Use the power of visualization daily to visualize your whole body as radiant with vibrant glowing positive health.

Yoga also teaches us to listen to our symptoms, as these are the body's way of telling us that it is unhappy with its current treatment. Frequently, by making the necessary life style changes, aches and pains start to melt away. But there are some routines that are of particular use when we are suffering from specific symptoms. In the table on page 174 I give my favourite prescriptions for some of the most widespread modern maladies.

Yoga and Pregnancy

I recommend yoga practise throughout pregnancy. However, as the pregnancy progresses it is important to have your medical practitioner's go-ahead, as well as guidance from a trained yoga teacher as movements have to be altered to cope with the increasing size of your baby. In general, if you have no history of miscarriage and have been practising yoga regularly prior to becoming pregnant, there is no reason why you should not continue. Avoid all movements that put strain on the abdomen – the Pose of a Cobra, the Locust Positions, the Pose of a Bow, the Salute to the Sun, the Pose of a Dog, the Pose of a Boat, Abdominal Lift and Contractions are all forbidden, as are the Spinal Twists, the Shoulder Stand and the Headstand. Yoga breathing and relaxation techniques are most beneficial. The Pose of a Cat (see page 88) is excellent for relieving lower backache and the Thigh Stretch (see page 78) is great for ensuring flexibility in the hip joints.

If you have never practised yoga before and would like to start yoga in pregnancy, wait until after your 15th week of pregnancy. With your medical practitioner's permission and a good teacher, yoga will help both your pregnancy and labour.

Enjoy your pregnancy, learn to relax, stay calm, listen to beautiful music. Peaceful relaxed mums make happy, calm babies.

[Note: Although yoga is extremely beneficial to your health, it must never by used as a substitute for treatment by a qualified medical practitioner. Before doing the recommended movements please ask your practitioner for permission and find a qualified yoga teacher to help and guide you.]

Health Problem	Exercise	Beneficial Effects
ARTHRITIS AND RHEUMATISM	Start each day with a Ten-minute Miracle (page 3).	To keep the spine flexible
	Arm Exercises (Chp. 6);	Ensuring maximum flexibility in the shoulders
	Alternate Leg Pull (page 76); Thigh Stretch (page 78).	Helping your hips, knees and ankles
ASTHMA	Start each day with a Ten-minute Miracle (page 3).	To relieve tension from the spine
	Alternate Nostril Breathing (page 95);	Keeping your stress levels down
	Also try: Backwards Bend (page 50); Pose of a Camel (page 91); Pose of a Cobra (page 87); The Wheel (page 126);	Helping to relieve tightness in the chest
	End each day with the Pose of a Fish (page 99).	To open and free the chest
BACK PROBLEMS	Start each day with a Ten-minute Miracle (page 3).	The spine has 6 areas of movement and this brilliant sequence works the spine all 6 ways
	Pose of a Cat (page 88); Back Rock at the end of the Pose of a Boat (page 56); Pose of a Heron (page 48)	To relieve tension from the spine To soothe the spine To strengthen the lower back Stretches the hamstrings

Health Problem	Exercise	Beneficial Effects
TENSION AND HEADACHES	The Chest Expansion (page 62); Pose of a Cow (page 70); The Mountain Pose (page 68); Pose of a Rabbit (page 94); Head and Neck Exercises (page 96).	Releasing tension in the neck and shoulders To relieve pressure from the shoulders To relieve neck tension To relieve neck tension and to keep the neck flexible
INSOMNIA	Before you go to bed: Pose of a Cat (page 88); Pose of a Cobra (page 87); Locust Positions (page 43); Pose of a Bow (page 117); Back Stretch (page 82); Slow Motion Firming (page 58); Complete Breath (page 62)	We carry a lot of our tension in the spine and these brilliant movements relieve this tension and helps us to feel calm and peaceful To calm the mind
PREMENSTRUAL TENSION	Start each day with a Ten-minute Miracle (page 3).	To relieve tension
	Daily, except during your period: Pose of a Cobra (page 87); Locust Positions (page 43); Pose of a Bow (page 117).	These movements greatly relieve tension in the abdominal region
REPETITIVE STRESS INJURY	Start each day with a Ten-minute Miracle (page 3). Arm Exercises (Chp. 6). The Mountain Pose (page 68); The Chest Expansion (page 62); Pose of a Cow (page 70); Head and Neck Exercises (page 96).	To help keep the spine tension free All these movement free the neck and shoulders from the tension resulting from overuse of the arms

And Finally ...

I do hope that I have helped you understand the value and benefits of yoga in your life. Keep practicing often and you will do more for your body, mind, health, and feelings of well-being than you ever thought possible.

With my love

Barbara Currie

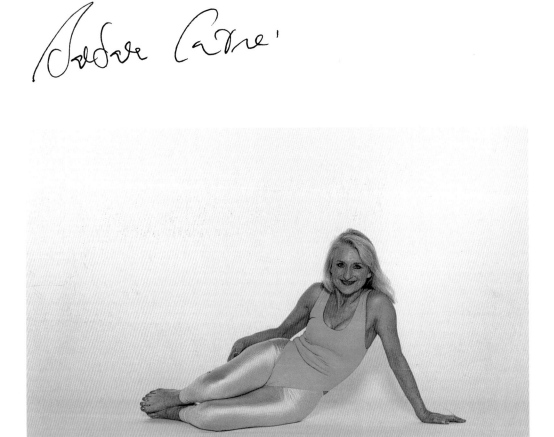

Let the waters settle you will see stars and moon mirrored in your being.

RUMI